ENT

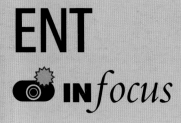

IN *focus*

D1100118

Robin Youngs MD FRCS
Consultant ENT Surgeon
Gloucestershire Royal Hospital
Gloucester, UK

Nicholas D Stafford MBChB FRCS
Professor of Otolaryngology and Head and Neck Surgery
University of Hull School of Medicine
Hull, UK

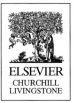

ELSEVIER
CHURCHILL
LIVINGSTONE

EDINBURGH   LONDON   NEW YORK   OXFORD   PHILADELPHIA   ST LOUIS   SYDNEY   TORONTO 2005

ELSEVIER
CHURCHILL
LIVINGSTONE

An imprint of Elsevier Limited

© Longman Group UK Limited 1994
© Harcourt Publishers Limited 1999
© 2005, Elsevier Limited. All rights reserved.

First published as Colour Aids—ENT 1988
Published as Colour Guide—ENT 1994
Second Colour Guide edition 1999
First In Focus edition 2005

ISBN 0443100802

British Library Cataloguing in Publication Data
A catalogue record for this book is available from the British Library

Library of Congress Cataloging in Publication Data
A catalog record for this book is available from the Library of Congress

Note
Medical knowledge is constantly changing. Standard safety precautions must be followed, but as new research and clinical experience broaden our knowledge, changes in treatment and drug therapy may become necessary or appropriate. Readers are advised to check the most current product information provided by the manufacturer of each drug to be administered to verify the recommended dose, the method and duration of administration, and contraindications. It is the responsibility of the practitioner, relying on experience and knowledge of the patient, to determine dosages and the best treatment for each individual patient. Neither the publisher nor the authors assumes any liability for any injury and/or damage to persons or property arising from this publication.

**your source for books,
journals and multimedia
in the health sciences**

www.elsevierhealth.com

The
publisher's
policy is to use
**paper manufactured
from sustainable forests**

Printed in China

Acknowledgements

The authors are very grateful to the Department of Medical Photography at St Mary's Hospital, London, and the Departments of Medical Illustration at St Bartholomew's Hospital, London, and Ipswich Hospital for their help in obtaining material for the book. Thanks also to Mr J Wright (Figs 52, 64 and 87), Dr A Choy (Figs 35 and 41), Dr T Lissauer (Figs 106, 140 and 156), Mr D Archer (Figs 95 and 165), Mr N Breach (Fig. 13), Mr D Davies (Fig. 160), Mr J Eyre (Fig. 116), Dr A Forge (Fig. 54), Dr J M Henk (Fig. 120) and Mr P Rhys-Evans (Fig. 121). The authors particularly appreciate the generosity of Professor Michael Hawke in offering them the use of some of his excellent tele-otoscopic pictures (Figs 9, 15, 17, 23, 27 and 34). Finally, the authors wish to express their gratitude to the patients appearing in this book, without whose cooperation this work would not have been possible.

Cheltenham and Hull   RY
2004   NDS

Contents

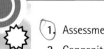

INfocus Contents

Otoscopy

The external ear should be inspected for abnormalities, which may include scars from previous middle ear surgery. The external ear canal is S-shaped and can be straightened by upward and backward traction on the pinna, giving a good view of the tympanic membrane in most cases (Fig. 1). The normal tympanic membrane has a grey, translucent appearance with the handle of the malleus visible centrally (Fig. 2). The lower part of the membrane is very thin and is known as the pars tensa. In the upper part the skin is thicker and is known as the pars flaccida.

Tuning fork tests

A 512 Hz tuning fork can be used to crudely assess hearing (Fig. 3). Using the Rinne and Weber tests, a diagnosis of conductive deafness due to middle ear disease can be distinguished from sensorineural deafness due to inner ear disease.

Audiometry

Pure tone audiometry is used to measure the threshold of hearing across a range of frequencies (Fig. 4). Impedance audiometry measures the compliance of the tympanic membrane in response to changing pressure in the ear canal. In this way middle ear pressure and the presence of middle ear fluid can be assessed.

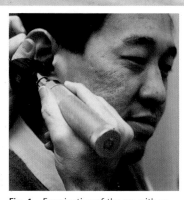

Fig. 1 Examination of the ear with an otoscope.

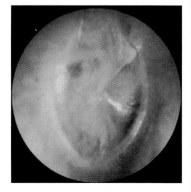

Fig. 2 Normal tympanic membrane.

(grey, translucent appearance
– handle of malleus visible centrally)

pars flaccida

pars tensa

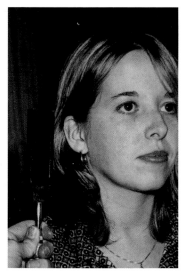

Fig. 3 Rinne's tuning fork test of hearing.

512Hz tuning fork.

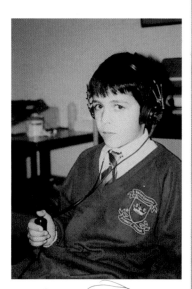

Fig. 4 Pure tone audiometry.

2 Congenital ear disease

External ear

Clinical features

The pinna may be absent or rudimentary (microtia) (Fig. 5). Failure of obliteration of the first branchial cleft results in a congenital sinus usually found in front of the helix or tragus (Fig. 6), which may become a site of infection requiring its excision. Accessory auricles can occur adjacent to a normally placed pinna (Fig. 7).

Middle ear

Clinical features

Ossicular chain defects often occur in association with atresia of the external auditory canal. Treacher–Collins syndrome consists of middle and external ear malformation with abnormal facial bone development.

Management

Bone anchored hearing aids and auricular prostheses (Fig. 8) have greatly improved the treatment of these conditions. particularly in bilateral cases. With this technique prostheses are secured directly to the bones of the skull via osseo-integrated screws passing through the skin.

Inner ear

Congenital defects of the inner ear usually result in severe sensorineural deafness. These disorders may have a hereditary basis. Damage to the inner ear can also be caused by events during pregnancy and the perinatal period. These include infections, particularly maternal rubella and syphilis, haemolytic disease of the newborn and fetal anoxia during birth.

Management

In the management of congenital ear disease it is vital that deafness, if present, is detected at an early stage so that treatment is instituted, allowing optimum language development during early childhood.

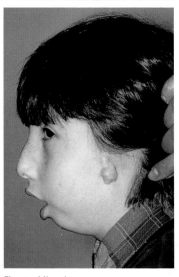

Fig. 5 Microtia.

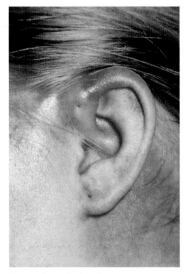

Fig. 6 Preauricular sinus.

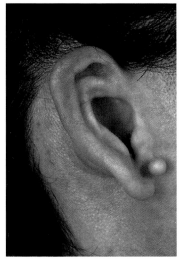

Fig. 7 Accessory auricles.

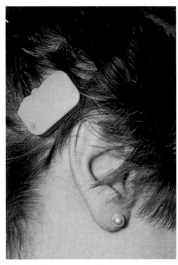

Fig. 8 Bone anchored hearing aid in place.

Foreign bodies

Clinical features

Foreign bodies are most commonly found in children, e.g. beads, cotton wool buds (Fig. 9). If deeply inserted into the external ear canal, they may cause tympanic membrane perforation (Fig. 10).

Management

Removal of foreign bodies may require a general anaesthetic. Most traumatic tympanic membrane perforations heal spontaneously.

Cauliflower ear

Clinical features

Blunt trauma to the pinna may produce a subperichondrial haematoma (Fig. 11). Devoid of its blood supply, the cartilage necroses and is replaced by fibrous tissue, resulting in an ugly cosmetic deformity (Fig. 12).

Management

Early drainage of the haematoma usually prevents any deformity.

Perichondritis

Perichondritis may result from open trauma, which may be surgical, involving the cartilage of the pinna or auditory meatus. Occasionally it complicates a severe otitis externa.

Clinical features

Presents as a generalized red, painful and tender swelling of the pinna and oedema may also stenose the meatus. A severe facial cellulitis and necrosis of the cartilage may develop.

Management

Treatment is with antibiotics and surgical drainage of any abscess.

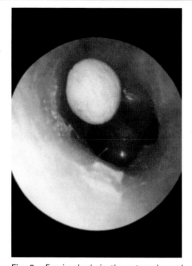

Fig. 9   Foreign body in the external canal.

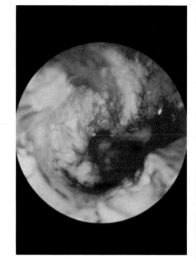

Fig. 10   Traumatic perforation.

— if deep → tympanic membrane perforation

blunt trauma → subperichondrial haematoma → cartilage necroses → fibrous tissue) ugly cosmetic deformity!

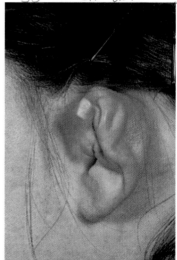

Fig. 11   Subperichondrial haematoma due to trauma.

Fig. 12   Cauliflower ear.

4 Tumours of the pinna and external auditory meatus

Malignant tumours

BCC   SCC

Basal cell carcinomas, squamous cell carcinomas (Fig. 13) and malignant melanomas occur on the skin of the pinna. Exposure to sunlight over a long period is a major risk factor.

Clinical features

Initially small superficial lesions progressing to deep ulceration in advanced cases. Squamous carcinomas and malignant melanomas metastasize to regional cervical lymph nodes.

Management

Treated by surgical excision, although radiotherapy is an alternative for basal and squamous carcinomas. Involvement of cartilage renders the tumour less radiosensitive.

Benign tumours

Bony swellings of the external auditory meatus are most common.

Aetiology

Osteomas are solitary and are true benign neoplasms. **Exostoses** are usually multiple, being associated with repeated exposure of the external auditory canal to cold water as in swimming or diving.

Clinical features

Present as smooth swellings on the wall of the bony meatus (Fig. 14). They are often asymptomatic but, if the lumen of the meatus is occluded, retention of wax, otitis externa or hearing loss may occur.

Management

None if asymptomatic. If recurrent otitis externa occurs, osteomas may be surgically reduced.

exostoses - multiple
osteomas - solitary

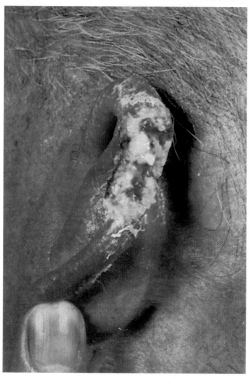

Fig. 13 Squamous carcinoma of the pinna.

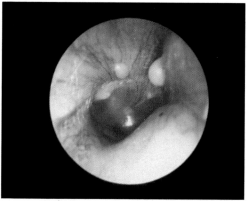

Fig. 14 Exostoses of the external auditory canal.

5 Otitis externa

Definition	Inflammation of the skin of the external auditory meatus.
Aetiology	Caused by either primary infection or contact sensitivity to topically applied substances such as cosmetics or antibiotics. Gram-negative organisms (e.g. *Proteus*, *Pseudomonas*) and fungi (e.g. *Aspergillus*) are often found. Precipitating factors include impacted cerumen, local trauma, middle ear discharge through a tympanic membrane perforation, swimming and skin conditions such as psoriasis and seborrhoeic dermatitis.
Clinical features	Presents as otalgia, otorrhoea and deafness. The skin of the external auditory meatus is oedematous and inflamed (Figs 15 & 16). The meatus may be occluded with discharge and in fungal infections hypae may be seen (Fig. 17). Traction on the pinna increases the otalgia, a sign not found in inflammatory conditions of the middle ear.
Management	Debris must be removed from the meatus, either by dry mopping or by suction aided by the use of an operating microscope. A swab of the meatus is taken for bacteriology prior to the instillation of drops containing an antibiotic and steroid mixture. If the meatus is totally occluded, an impregnated gauze wick may be inserted. In severe cases with cellulitis spreading onto the pinna (Fig. 18) systemic antibiotics are also needed.

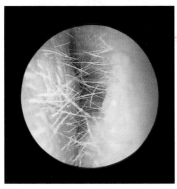

Fig. 15 Otitis externa with canal wall oedema.

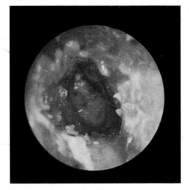

Fig. 16 Bacterial otitis externa.

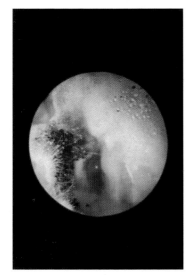

Fig. 17 Fungal otitis externa.

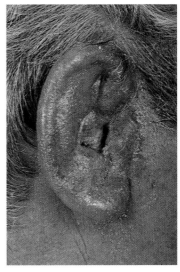

Fig. 18 Cellulitis of the pinna secondary to otitis externa.

Furunculosis of the external auditory meatus

Staphylococcal infection of hair follicles found in the lateral part of the meatus.

Clinical features

Presents as severe otalgia exacerbated by traction on the pinna, with deafness if the meatus becomes occluded. The furuncle is often visible.

Management

Most furuncles rupture spontaneously. Ribbon gauze impregnated with glycerin/ichthammol may be inserted daily into the meatus (Fig. 19). Systemic flucloxacillin and analgesics are also needed.

Necrotizing (malignant) otitis externa

A potentially fatal *Pseudomonas* infection of the external auditory meatus, with spread to the skull base. It occurs in elderly diabetics and also in patients with HIV/AIDS.

Clinical features

Presents as severe otalgia, otorrhoea and deafness with progression to cranial nerve palsies (VII, IX, X, XI, XII) in advanced cases.

Management

Treatment is by local surgery, usually mastoidectomy, combined with a prolonged course of specific anti-pseudomonal antibiotics. Skull base involvement and its response to treatment may be assessed by radioisotope scanning (Fig. 20).

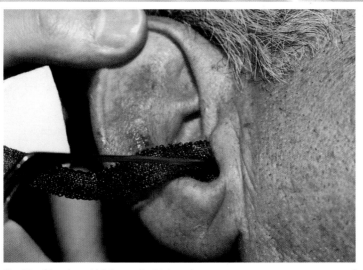

Fig. 19 Glycerin and <u>ichthammol</u> wick insertion.

↳ daily into
meatus
+ sy

ichthammol
ichthammol

glycerin)
ichthammol
wick

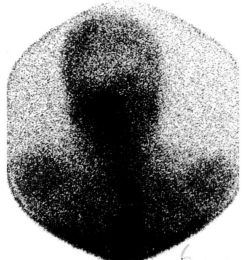

Fig. 20 Gallium scan in necrotizing otitis externa:
increased uptake at petrous apex.

Bullous myringitis

Aetiology

An influenza virus infection of the tympanic membrane and deep external meatus, often associated with an acute otitis media.

Clinical features

Presents as otalgia, deafness and serosanguinous otorrhoea. Haemorrhagic bullae are seen on otoscopy (Fig. 21). Secondary bacterial infection can occur with purulent otorrhoea leading to otitis externa.

Management

Treat with analgesics; local and systemic antibiotics for secondary bacterial infection.

Tympanosclerosis

Aetiology

Deposits of collagen beneath the mucosa of the tympanic membrane and middle ear following otitis media or middle ear surgery, particularly grommet insertion.

Clinical features

Tympanosclerosis is mostly asymptomatic. Deposits are visible as white 'chalk patches' in the tympanic membrane (Fig. 22). Middle ear deposits may cause conductive deafness by ossicular fixation.

Management

None if asymptomatic. Ossiculoplasty may be required for conductive deafness.

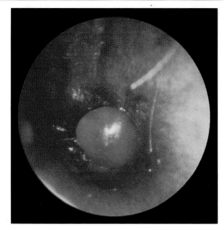

Fig. 21 Bullous myringitis.

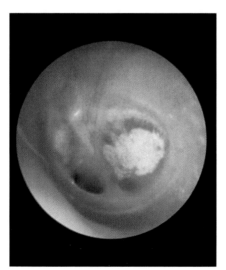

Fig. 22 Tympanosclerosis of the tympanic membrane.

7 Middle ear effusions 'Glue Ear'

Aetiology

Middle ear effusion is often associated with Eustachian tube obstruction, either acute during upper respiratory infections or chronic as in childhood adenoid hypertrophy. In adults middle ear effusions may result from Eustachian tube obstruction by a nasopharyngeal neoplasm. Changes in atmospheric pressure occurring during flight or diving may also result in effusions: otitic barotrauma.

Incidence

Middle ear effusion is a common paediatric problem, particularly in the 4–7 age group.

Clinical features

On otoscopy the tympanic membrane is dull with a loss of light reflex (Fig. 23). Small vessels are often seen radiating from the handle of the malleus and occasionally a fluid level is seen (Fig. 24). Deafness in children may lead to poor language development and educational performance. Diagnosis may be confirmed by impedance audiometry in which the compliance of the tympanic membrane is measured in response to pressure changes in the external auditory meatus.

Management

Medical treatment: consists of the use of topical and systemic decongestants.

Surgical treatment: consists of myringotomy and insertion of a ventilation tube into the affected tympanic membrane (Figs 25 & 26). Children may also require an adenoidectomy whilst in adults a nasopharyngeal tumour must be excluded.

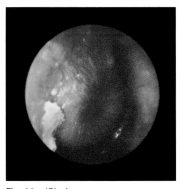

Fig. 23 'Glue' ear.

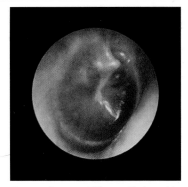

Fig. 24 Serous middle ear effusion with fluid level.

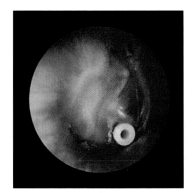

Fig. 25 Grommet in situ.

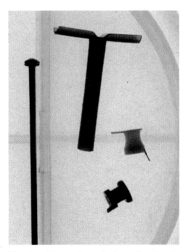

Fig. 26 Types of ventilation tube: Goode T tube, Shah and Sheppard grommets (top to bottom).

8 Suppurative otitis media

Acute otitis media

Aetiology

Acute infection of the middle ear cleft, common in young children. This usually occurs as part of an upper respiratory tract infection, with *Haemophilus influenzae* and *Pneumococcus* being the most common pathogens.

Clinical features

Presents as severe otalgia and deafness. The tympanic membrane is red and bulging (Fig. 27). Rupture may occur leading to purulent otorrhoea.

Management

Treat with oral antibiotic therapy (amoxicillin, co-trimoxazole or erythromycin) and adequate analgesia.

Acute mastoiditis

Aetiology

Acute mastoiditis may complicate acute otitis media. Infection of the mastoid air cell system occurs.

Clinical features

Presents as worsening of otalgia with tenderness over the mastoid antrum. The external meatus may be narrowed by oedema of the posterior–superior wall. In advanced cases a subperiosteal abscess may push the ear forward (Fig. 28). Diagnosis is confirmed by opacity of the mastoid cells on CT scan (Fig. 29).

Management

Initially high-dose parenteral antibiotic therapy is required, although in cases that fail to respond to antibiotics, or in which a subperiosteal abscess has formed, surgical drainage via a cortical mastoidectomy is required.

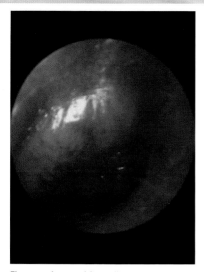

Fig. 27 Acute otitis media.

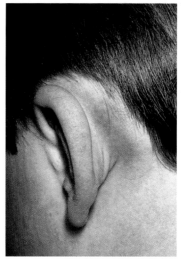

Fig. 28 Postauricular swelling and redness in acute mastoiditis.

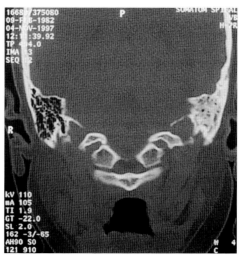

Fig. 29 CT scan showing mastoid opacity in mastoiditis.

Chronic otitis media

Aetiology

Chronic inflammation of the middle ear cleft is usually associated with a perforation of the tympanic membrane. Perforations usually result from previous episodes of acute otitis media when the membrane fails to heal following rupture, but can be due to direct or indirect trauma. In children, perforations can persist following extrusion of ventilation tubes from the tympanic membrane. Organisms can reach the middle ear from the Eustachian tube or from the external meatus. Chronic middle ear infection is also associated with ossicular damage, with the incudostapedial joint being the most commonly affected linkage.

Clinical features

A *central perforation* in the pars tensa part of the membrane (Figs 30 & 31) is associated with recurrent otorrhoea and conductive deafness. This type of perforation is regarded as 'safe' as neurological complications are rare. An *attic* or *marginal perforation* (Fig. 32) can be associated with the development of a cholesteatoma and is regarded as 'unsafe'.

Management

Cases of central perforation should be kept dry. If recurrent otorrhoea occurs, ear drops containing a mixture of steroid and antibiotic are used and attention should be paid to possible sources of infection in the nasopharynx, nose and paranasal sinuses. A dry perforation can be repaired by myringoplasty. Traumatic central perforations usually heal spontaneously.

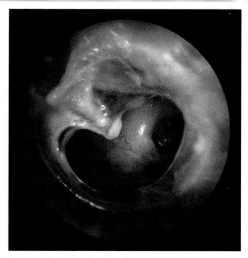

Fig. 30 Dry central perforation.

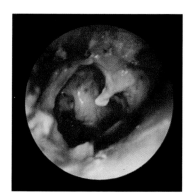

Fig. 31 Subtotal perforation.

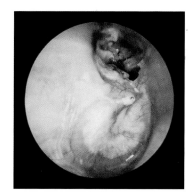

Fig. 32 Dry attic perforation.

9 Cholesteatoma

A ball of keratinizing stratified squamous epithelium in the middle ear cleft or mastoid which enlarges and can destroy or erode local structures. It is a feature of the 'unsafe' type of chronic middle ear disease.

Aetiology

The most widely accepted theory of its development is the immigration–retraction pocket theory: in response to Eustachian tube obstruction and negative middle ear pressure an inward retraction of the tympanic membrane occurs, usually in the attic region. Desquamated epithelium normally shed from the membrane into the meatus collects in the pocket, the continued enlargement of which results in the formation of a cholesteatoma sac. Congenital cholesteatoma is very rare (Fig. 33) and results from congenital squamous cell rests within the temporal bone.

Clinical features

Presents as progressive conductive hearing loss with purulent, and often offensive, otorrhoea. Pain or vertigo due to bony erosion may also occur. Otoscopy reveals a retraction pocket or perforation in the attic or posterior marginal region of the tympanic membrane (Fig. 34) with flaky white debris visible in the defect. Nystagmus and other evidence of neurological involvement should be sought.

Management

Radical mastoidectomy involves removal of the cholesteatoma, middle ear structures and bone of the bony external meatus, producing a smooth exteriorized mastoid cavity accessible for inspection. The operation may be modified in order to conserve hearing by retaining part of the ossicular chain and tympanic membrane (Fig. 35).

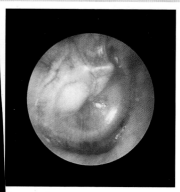

Fig. 33 Congenital cholesteatoma behind an intact tympanic membrane.

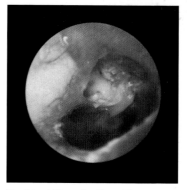

Fig. 34 Attic perforation with cholesteatoma.

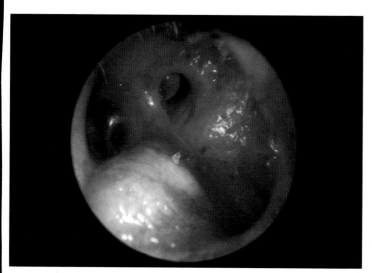

Fig. 35 Healed left modified radical mastoidectomy cavity.

10 Complications of suppurative otitis media

Extracranial

Facial nerve paralysis

Aetiology

Pressure by cholesteatoma on the facial nerve in the middle ear or mastoid.

Clinical features

Presents as partial or complete lower motor neurone facial paralysis (Fig. 36) with evidence of chronic middle ear disease on otoscopy.

Management

Treatment is by immediate surgical decompression of the facial nerve via a mastoidectomy operation.

Suppurative labyrinthitis

Aetiology

Follows erosion of the bony labyrinth most commonly over the lateral semicircular canal. In the early stages compression of the air in the external meatus causes vertigo from mechanical stimulation of the labyrinth (fistula test). Later purulent infection in the inner ear causes severe vertigo and sensorineural deafness.

Management

Treatment is by intravenous antibiotics and eradication of cholesteatoma via mastoidectomy.

Gradenigo's syndrome

Otorrhoea is associated with pain behind the eye and diplopia, caused by fifth and sixth nerve irritation resulting from air cell infection at the petrous apex (Fig. 37).

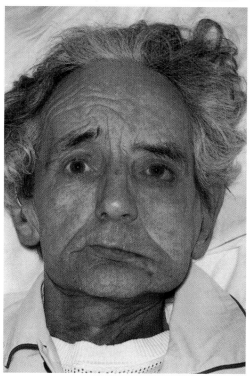

Fig. 36 Complete lower motor neurone facial palsy.

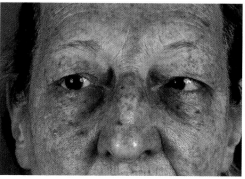

Fig. 37 Gradenigo's syndrome: patient looking to right.

Intracranial

Intracranial spread of organisms may occur via the middle ear by thrombophlebitis or by penetration of the dura of the middle or posterior cranial fossae.

Meningitis

Clinical features

Presents as headache, neck stiffness and photophobia. Lumbar puncture confirms the diagnosis. *Pneumococcus* and *Haemophilus influenzae* are common pathogens.

Management

Treatment is by intravenous antibiotics followed by mastoidectomy once the meningitis has resolved.

Venous sinus thrombosis

Follows spread of middle ear and mastoid infection through the bone over the sigmoid sinus.

Clinical features

Presents as headache, pyrexia and rigors. Extension of thrombus to the superior sagittal sinus leads to CSF outflow obstruction: otitic hydrocephalus.

Management

Treatment is by intravenous antibiotics and mastoidectomy, during which infected thrombus may need to be removed from the sinus lumen (Fig. 38).

Intracranial abscess

Extradural, subdural and cerebral abscesses occur. Infection spreads into the middle and posterior cranial fossae leading to temporal lobe and cerebellar abscesses respectively. Diagnosis is by CT scan (Figs 39 & 40) and treatment by neurosurgical drainage.

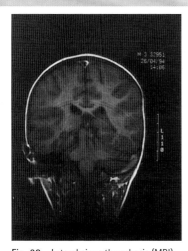

Fig. 38   Lateral sinus thrombosis (MRI).

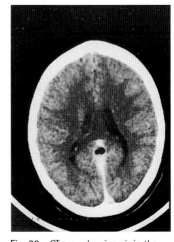

Fig. 39   CT scan showing air in the subdural space in a subdural abscess.

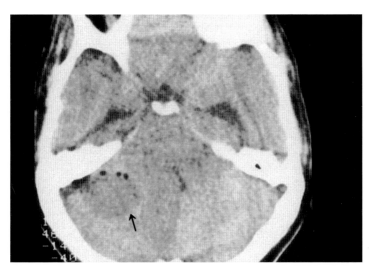

Fig. 40   Otogenic cerebellar abscess on CT scan.

A disease primarily of the bone of the otic capsule which causes a conductive hearing loss, usually because of stapes fixation. A sensorineural deafness may occur in the later stages.

Incidence

The disease is usually bilateral and presents between the ages of 15 and 45 years. Tinnitus is common and 25% of patients have positional vertigo. 70% have a family history of otosclerosis.

Clinical features

Examination of the tympanic membrane is usually normal, the pink drum (Schwartze sign) being rare and indicative of active disease (Fig. 41). In the early stages the audiogram shows a pure conductive loss, frequently with a Cahart's notch at 2000 Hz (Fig. 42).

Management

An air conduction hearing aid is frequently very successful for the patient. In the stapedotomy operation the stapes arch is replaced by a piston, usually made of Teflon (Fig. 43). Stapedotomy will produce excellent improvement in hearing level in the majority of cases, although profound deafness and vertigo are occasional complications.

A rare variant is seen in association with osteogenesis imperfecta (van der Hoeve syndrome), these patients being recognized by their blue sclera. Stapedectomy is less successful in these cases.

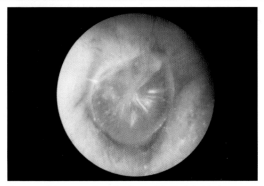

Fig. 41   Schwartze sign: flamingo pink flush behind tympanic membrane.

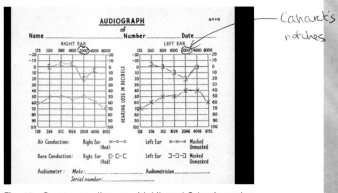

Cahart's notches

Fig. 42   Pure tone audiogram with bilateral Cahart's notches.

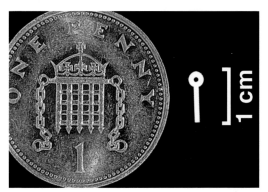

Fig. 43   Teflon stapes prosthesis.

Myringoplasty

Central perforations may be repaired when accompanied by deafness or recurrent middle ear infections, or when an intact tympanic membrane is required for swimming, or as a condition of employment. Fascia overlying the temporalis muscle is usually used (Fig. 44) and may be placed medial (underlay) or lateral (onlay) to the perforation.

Ossiculoplasty

Performed for conductive deafness where the ossicular chain has been interrupted by chronic infection, trauma or congenital deformity. Replacement ossicles may be constructed from natural or synthetic materials. Bone is the favoured material; where possible the patient's own incus remnant is remodelled and transposed.

Eradication of mastoid disease: mastoidectomy

Performed for acute mastoiditis failing to respond to high-dose antibiotics, otorrhoea due to chronic mastoid infection, and middle ear and mastoid cholesteatoma.

Cortical mastoidectomy: involves exenterating the mastoid air cell system without interfering with the external meatus, ossicles or tympanic membrane (Fig. 45).

Radical and modified radical mastoidectomy: for cholesteatoma involves removal of the posterior meatal wall, creating a large cavity accessible for cleaning (Fig. 46).

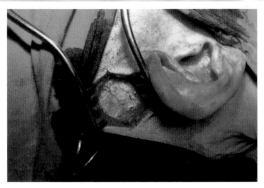

Fig. 44 Harvesting a temporalis fascia graft.

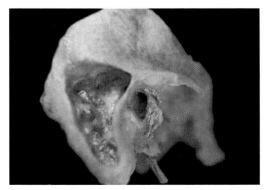

Fig. 45 Cortical mastoidectomy (cadaver dissection).
↳ only Mastoid air cells

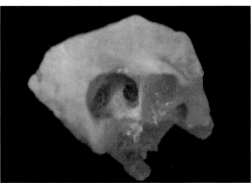

Fig. 46 Radical mastoidectomy (cadaver dissection). Everything out?
↳ Mastoid air cells, ossicles, External meatus & TM.

13 Facial nerve palsy

Disruption of the lower motor neurone facial nerve can occur at any point between its brainstem nucleus and the facial musculature.

Bell's (idiopathic) palsy

Clinical features

Most common palsy with no identifiable cause although a viral or vascular aetiology postulated. Palsy may be partial or complete.

Management

Total recovery occurs in 90% of cases. Treatment with steroids or surgical decompression controversial.

Ramsay Hunt syndrome

Clinical features

Herpes zoster involvement of the facial nerve with herpetic vesicles on the tympanic membrane (Fig. 47), pinna (Fig. 48) or palate. May present with severe otalgia alone. Auditory and trigeminal nerves may be affected.

Management

Recovers fully in about 60% of cases. If given early, the antiviral agent aciclovir may enhance recovery. The value of steroids or surgical decompression of the nerve remains unproven.

Temporal bone fracture

Clinical features

Longitudinal fractures (80%) are associated with a facial palsy in 20% of cases and a conductive deafness. Transverse fractures (20%) are associated with a facial palsy in 50% of cases and a sensorineural deafness. Diagnosis is confirmed by CT scan (Fig. 49).

Management

Exploration of the nerve may be indicated in cases of immediate, complete paralysis but is likely to be followed by deafness.

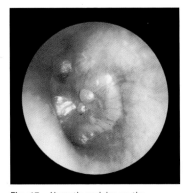

Fig. 47 Herpetic vesicles on the tympanic membrane.

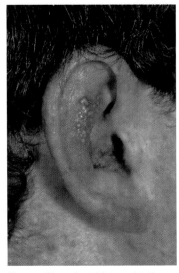

Fig. 48 Herpetic vesicles on the pinna.

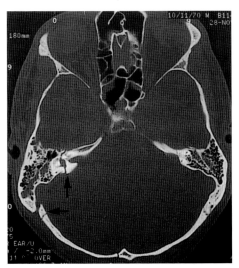

Fig. 49 Temporal bone fracture. (CT-scan).

Otogenic vertigo is an hallucination or a false sensation of movement. Disease affecting the vestibular apparatus may produce rotatory vertigo accompanied by horizontal nystagmus.

Testing

Caloric testing (Fig. 50). Involves stimulating the vestibular apparatus by irrigating the external meatus with water at varying temperatures; the duration of induced nystagmus is recorded, allowing comparison between the two sides.

Positional testing (Fig. 51). Vertigo provoked by head movements (positional vertigo) may be a feature of inner ear disease, cervical spondylosis or disease affecting central vestibular pathways in the brainstem.

Ménière's disease

Aetiology

Unknown; may be due to imbalance between production and absorption of inner ear endolymph or disturbance of inner ear immunity.

Clinical features

Episodic rotatory vertigo, tinnitus and sensorineural deafness may be present. Unilateral in early stages.

Management

Vestibular sedatives for acute attacks. Surgery may be conservative (endolymphatic sac decompression) or destructive (labyrinthectomy or vestibular neurectomy). Intratympanic gentamicin is also an option.

Sudden unilateral vestibular failure

Aetiology

Unknown aetiology. Viral infection, ischaemia and inner ear membrane rupture have been postulated.

Clinical features

Presents with sudden onset of vertigo. Recovery takes place by central compensation.

Management

Vestibular sedatives are useful in the acute phase.

Other causes of vertigo are syphilis, suppurative labyrinthitis, temporal fractures and ototoxic drugs.

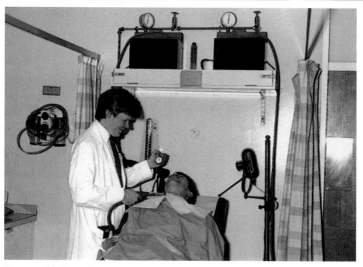

Fig. 50 Caloric testing.

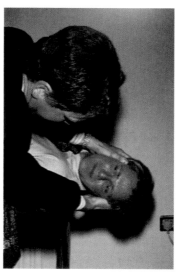

Fig. 51 Positional testing.

Sensorineural hearing loss results from disease in the cochlea or its central neuronal connections. The disease can be congenital (Fig. 52) or acquired.

Congenital

Aetiology

Aplasias. Partial or complete failure of inner ear development, e.g. Schiebe anomaly.

Abiotrophies. Inner ear anatomically developed but neural pathways degenerate prematurely, e.g. Pendred, Hurler and Alport syndromes.

Intrauterine/perinatal damage. Includes hypoxia, kernicterus, rubella, cytomegalovirus, syphilis, thalidomide.

Acquired

Aetiology

- Age-related presbyacusis: the most common
- Noise-induced hearing loss
- Ménière's disease
- Acoustic neuroma (Fig. 53)
- Trauma, e.g. head injury, middle ear surgery
- Sudden (idiopathic) sensorineural hearing loss
- Drug-induced hearing loss, e.g. gentamicin (Fig. 54)
- Syphilis/yaws.

Management

The management of any sensorineural hearing loss involves rehabilitation, once any treatable cause has been excluded. Special schooling may be necessary for the severely deaf child.

ménière's disease

↳disorder of the inner ear that can affect hearing & balance to a varying degree.

↳episodes of tinnitus & vertigo & progressive hearing loss, usually in one ear.

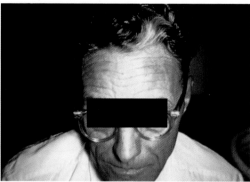

Fig. 52 White forelock in Waardenburg syndrome.

acustic neurome (vestibular schwannoma) ⇒ benign 1° intracranial tumour of myelin-forming cells of the CN VIII. (Vestibulo-cochlear nerve).

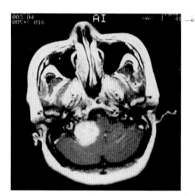

Fig. 53 Posterior fossa MRI scan showing an acoustic neuroma.

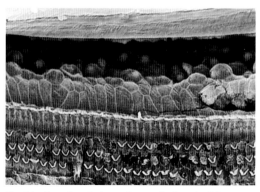

Fig. 54 Scanning electron micrograph of gentamicin-damaged cochlear hair cells.

Early diagnosis of deafness is the key to successful auditory rehabilitation, particularly in children with congenital deafness. With early intensive auditory training most children will develop the ability to communicate orally. Lip reading is an adjunct to oral communication. Manual communication, as in sign language, may be applicable for severely deaf people.

Hearing aids

Hearing aids amplify and modify incoming sound. The most modern aids use digital technology to tailor the performance of the aid to individual patterns of hearing loss. The postaural aid (Fig. 55) is most widely used, although body-worn and 'in the ear' alternatives exist (Fig. 56). Aids to communication such as electromagnetic 'loop' systems can enable hearing aids to function in a group environment such as a theatre or lecture hall.

Cochlear implants

Direct electrical stimulation of the cochlear portion of the inner ear in response to incoming sound waves has been investigated in the development of cochlear implants. Electrodes are either placed on the surface of the cochlea (extracochlear) or inserted into the lumen of the cochlea (intracochlear) (Fig. 57).

The use of cochlear implantation is now established in patients with both acquired and congenital severe sensorineural hearing loss. Profoundly deaf children ideally have implants fitted before primary school age.

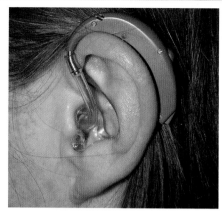

Fig. 55 Postaural hearing aid.

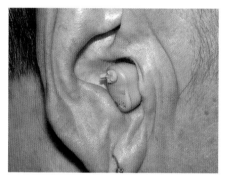

Fig. 56 An 'in the ear' hearing aid.

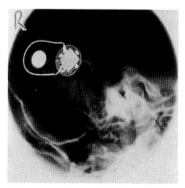

Fig. 57 X-ray showing cochlear implant in situ.

Nasal obstruction, rhinorrhoea, epistaxis or facial pain may indicate intranasal or paranasal sinus disease. Clinical assessment begins with observation. Is the patient an obligatory mouth breather? Look for an obvious external nasal deformity. The nasal airway is then assessed. In children, this is undertaken using a chrome tongue depressor held just below the nose whilst the child breathes (Fig. 58). Misting of the chrome indicates a patent airway. In adults the examiner's thumb is used to close one airway at a time, being careful not to apply any lateral pressure that could occlude both sides simultaneously.

The two nasal cavities are then examined in turn using a Thudicums nasal speculum. The anterior nasal septum is assessed along with evaluation of the lateral nasal walls (Fig. 59). Only the inferior and middle turbinates can be seen by anterior rhinoscopy. The nasal mucosa is also evaluated for evidence of rhinitis.

Finally, the nasopharynx is examined. A tongue depressor is used to allow mirror examination of the nasopharynx and Eustachian tube orifices. Alternatively, fibreoptic endoscopy can be employed.

Depending on the suspected pathology, the ears, larynx and neck should also be assessed.

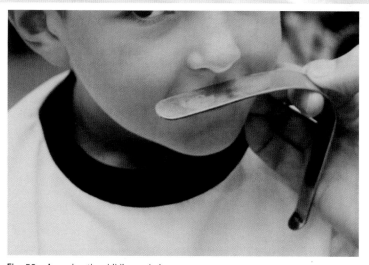

Fig. 58 Assessing the child's nasal airway.

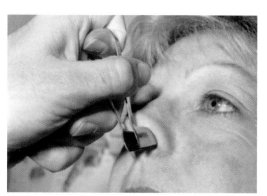

Fig. 59 Examining the nasal cavities.

Rhinophyma

Clinical features

Red nodular masses centred around the nasal tip in association with acne rosacea (Fig. 60), usually seen in elderly men.

Management

If unsightly, treat by dermabrasion or surgical shaving.

Lupus vulgaris

Aetiology

Inoculation of the bacterium *Mycobacterium tuberculosis*, possibly through nose picking.

Clinical features

Red/brown patches or nodules on the nasal or facial skin. Perforation of the cartilaginous nasal septum can occur, with scarring in long-standing cases (Fig. 61).

Management

Treatment is by antituberculous chemotherapy.

Lupus pernio

Clinical features

Skin lesions other than erythema nodosum occur in 20% of patients with sarcoidosis. Lupus pernio (Fig. 62) is common and is frequently associated with bone cysts and chest disease.

Management

Treat the underlying disease.

Malignant tumours

Clinical features

Basal or squamous cell carcinomas (Fig. 63) present as warty or ulcerating lesions, rarely with lymphadenopathy. Melanomas are more rare.

Management

Excision biopsy when possible; radiotherapy for larger tumours not involving bone.

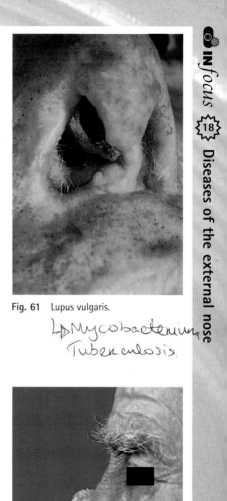

INfocus 18 Diseases of the external nose

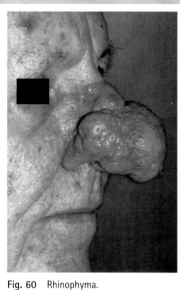

Fig. 60 Rhinophyma.

Fig. 61 Lupus vulgaris.

↳ Mycobacterium Tuberculosis

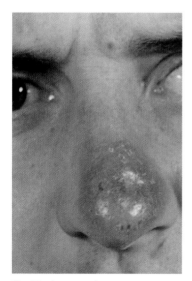

Fig. 62 Lupus pernio.

↳ Sarcoidosis skin manifestation

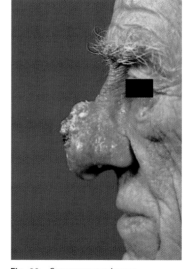

Fig. 63 Squamous carcinoma.

Aetiology

Most cases of epistaxis are idiopathic, although bleeding can also result from a number of specific conditions.

Local conditions include nasal trauma, nasal and paranasal sinus tumours and nasal septal perforations.

General conditions include systemic bleeding diatheses such as leukaemia, anticoagulant therapy and thrombocytopenia, and systemic vascular disorders. In hereditary haemorrhagic telangiectasia (Rendu–Osler–Weber syndrome, Fig. 64), epistaxis is a prominent feature and usually arises from abnormal vessels on the nasal septum.
   Systemic hypertension, although not a cause of epistaxis, is often associated with an increased severity of bleeding.

Clinical features

In most cases of epistaxis bleeding originates from the nasal septum, particularly Little's area just behind the mucocutaneous junction where there is a rich anastomosis of vessels (Kiesselbach's plexus, Fig. 65). Bleeding from a postero-superior site in the nasal cavity can occur, especially in the elderly. Haemorrhage can present via the anterior nares or pass backwards via the nasopharynx where it is spat out or swallowed. In severe cases with profuse blood loss, hypotension and tachycardia may occur.

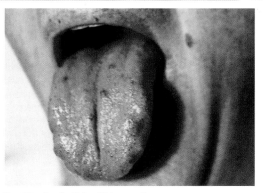

Fig. 64 Rendu–Osler–Weber syndrome.

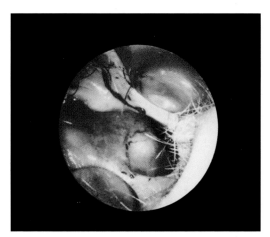

Fig. 65 Endoscopic view of prominent blood vessels in Little's area.

Management

Initial measures to stop bleeding consist of exerting pressure on Little's area by pinching the nose, with the patient leaning forward and spitting any blood into a bowl (Fig. 66). If a bleeding vessel is seen, it may be coagulated with chemical or electric cautery following topical application of local anaesthetic, but this is rarely successful in the acute stage. Epistaxis not responding to pressure necessitates nasal packing either with gauze impregnated with an antiseptic such as bismuth, iodoform and paraffin paste (BIPP) (Fig. 67) or with nasal balloons. Patients requiring nasal packing also require hospitalization.

In severe cases arterial ligation may be required. Endoscopic ligation or diathermy of the sphenopalatine artery in the nasal cavity is the commonest method. Other available arteries are the external carotid via the neck (Fig. 68) and the anterior ethmoidal via an inner canthal incision.

An alternative to arterial ligation in severe cases is arterial embolization performed with angiographic control by a radiologist. Intravenous resuscitation with blood or plasma substitute is necessary in cases where hypotension and tachycardia are present.

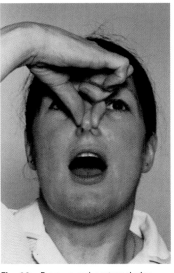

Fig. 66 Pressure and posture during epistaxis.

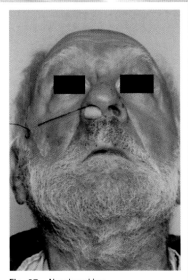

Fig. 67 Nasal packing.

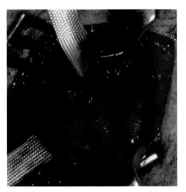

Fig. 68 External carotid artery just prior to ligation.

Deviated nasal septum

Aetiology

This occurs following previous nasal trauma or results from asymmetric septal development possibly following birth trauma.

Clinical features

Presents as unilateral nasal obstruction (Fig. 69) and less commonly epistaxis. The inferior and middle turbinates on the side opposite the septal deflection often undergo compensatory hypertrophy.

Management

If symptoms warrant, the septum can be positioned in the midline as in the operations of septoplasty and submucosal resection.

Septal haematoma

A collection of blood beneath the mucoperichondrium and posteriorly the mucoperiosteum of the nasal septum.

Aetiology

Usually complicates nasal trauma, either accidental or iatrogenic following septal surgery. Rarely a spontaneous haematoma can occur in a bleeding diathesis.

Clinical features

Presents as nasal obstruction with widening of the septum on inspection (Fig. 70).

Management

In the acute stage, treat by incision and drainage; however, after 48 h, organization of haematoma occurs and evacuation of the clot is difficult. Antibiotics are given to prevent secondary infection.

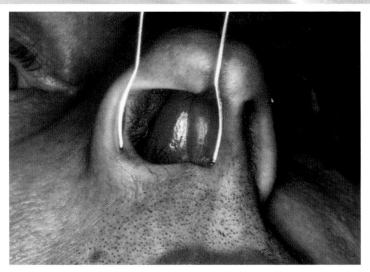

Fig. 69   Deviated nasal septum.

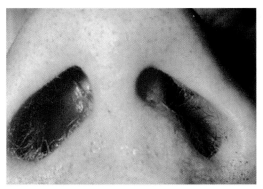

Fig. 70   Septal haematoma.

Septal abscess

Aetiology

Septal abscesses usually result from secondary infection of a septal haematoma.

Clinical features

Manifests by the development of severe pain, nasal swelling and pyrexia following a septal haematoma. Cartilage necrosis often complicates septal haematoma and abscess with the production of a saddle-nose deformity (Fig. 71).

Management

Treatment is by incision and drainage with appropriate antibiotic therapy.

Septal perforation

Aetiology

Traumatic: after septal surgery, nose picking, cocaine sniffing and pressure from foreign bodies and nasal polyps.

Infective: due to syphilis and tuberculosis.

Chronic inflammatory. Wegener's granulomatosis is a non-neoplastic upper airways granuloma associated with focal lung and kidney lesions. (Lethal) midline granuloma is thought to be an atypical lymphoma occurring in the midline of the face.

Clinical features

Asymptomatic, or nasal crusting and epistaxis are characteristic of septal perforation (Fig. 72).

Management

Treatment is by removal of crusts, nasal douches and treatment of underlying systemic conditions.

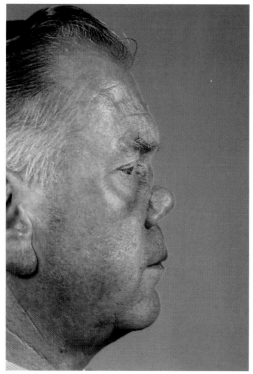

Fig. 71 Saddle-nose deformity following septal abscess.

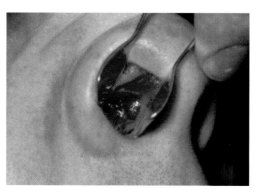

Fig. 72 Septal perforation.

Allergic rhinitis

Aetiology

Hypersensitivity to inhaled or ingested allergens causes nasal mucosal oedema and exudation. Allergy may be seasonal (e.g. pollens) or perennial (e.g. house dust). Allergies may be demonstrated by skin tests (Fig. 73).

Clinical features

Presents as nasal obstruction, sneezing and rhinorrhoea with mucosal oedema on examination (Fig. 74).

Management

Treat with steroid nasal spray and oral antihistamines. Avoid any known allergens.

Non-allergic rhinitis

Clinical features

Presents as chronic nasal obstruction and rhinorrhoea with no demonstrable allergy.

Management

If medical treatment in the form of antihistamines or steroid sprays fails to produce relief, nasal obstruction may be helped by surgical reduction or diathermy of the inferior turbinates.

Long term use of sympathomimetic vasoconstrictor nasal sprays can result in chronic nasal congestion as a rebound effect: rhinitis medicamentosa.

Atrophic rhinitis

Aetiology

A disease of unknown aetiology, occurring mainly in developing countries. It can occur following radical turbinectomy operations or radiotherapy to the nasal cavity.

Clinical features

Nasal crusting, anosmia and fetor are present. Paradoxically, although the nasal cavity is widely patent, the sensation of nasal obstruction is common.

Management

Treatment is by removal of crusts and nasal douches.

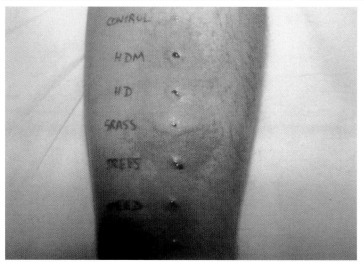

Fig. 73 Positive skin tests in allergic rhinitis.

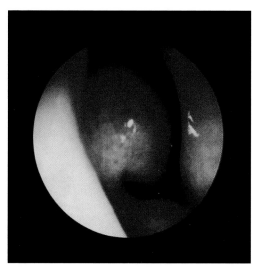

Fig. 74 Inferior turbinate hypertrophy.

22 Simple nasal polyps

Aetiology

Simple nasal polyps are pedunculated areas of oedematous mucosa occurring in the nasal cavity and paranasal sinuses. Their aetiology is unknown although chronic sinus infection and mucosal allergy have been suggested. Most polyps arise from the ethmoid sinuses with the maxillary antrum being a less common source.

Nasal polyps can be associated with asthma and aspirin sensitivity (aspirin triad). In children, nasal polyps may be a manifestation of cystic fibrosis.

Samters triad

Clinical features

Presents as progressive nasal obstruction and rhinorrhoea. On inspection of the nasal cavity, polyps are seen as pale grey, smooth swellings, which can fill the nasal cavity (Fig. 75). Most cases are bilateral but in unilateral cases a neoplasm must be excluded by biopsy. An antrochoanal polyp passes from the maxillary sinus via its ostium posteriorly into the nasal cavity to occupy the posterior choana where it can be seen on posterior rhinoscopy (Fig. 76) and its presence confirmed by lateral radiography.

Management

Medical treatment: topical steroid drops or spray administered correctly can cause considerable diminution in polyp size.

Surgical treatment: intranasal polypectomy (Fig. 77) may have to be repeated as recurrence after polyp removal is common. Many surgeons use endoscopic ethmoidectomy techniques to remove polyps from the ethmoid sinuses.

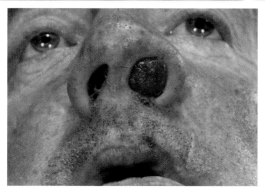

Fig. 75 Simple nasal polyps.

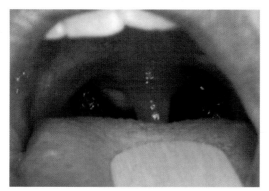

Fig. 76 Antrochoanal polyp behind soft palate.

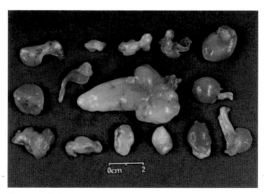

Fig. 77 Operative specimens from one patient.

Aetiology	Stasis and acute infection of sinus secretions may result from any pathological or anatomical abnormality obstructing free sinus drainage. The common cold is the most frequent cause. Acute maxillary sinusitis can also result from apical infection of an upper tooth root. The causative organism is usually *Pneumococcus, Streptococcus viridans* or *Haemophilus influenzae.*
Complications	Left untreated, acute sinusitis can rarely lead to orbital cellulitis, cavernous sinus thrombosis or intracranial abscess formation (Fig. 78). Chronic sinusitis is a far more common sequela.

Maxillary sinusitis

Clinical features	Most common type overall. Facial or dental pain may occur, as may referred otalgia. Nasal obstruction and purulent rhinorrhoea are also frequent. Local tenderness may be the only physical sign. An occipitomental X-ray usually shows a fluid level on one or both sides (Fig. 79), but this investigation is increasingly being replaced by CT scanning (Fig. 80).
Management	Treat with antibiotics and topical nasal decongestants. An antral washout (Fig. 81) through the inferior meatus may be necessary if resolution with antibiotics does not occur, but this form of treatment is decreasing in popularity with the advent of endoscopic management of sinusitis.

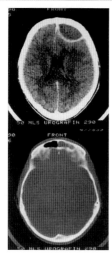

Fig. 78 Anterior fossa extradural abscess (upper scan) secondary to frontal sinusitis (lower scan).

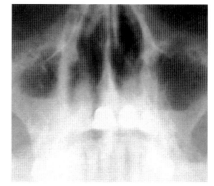

Fig. 79 Bilateral antral fluid levels.

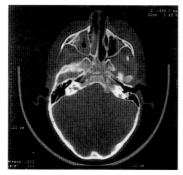

Fig. 80 CT scan of maxillary sinusitis.

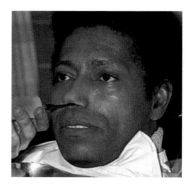

Fig. 81 Antral washout.

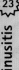

Ethmoiditis

Incidence

Most common in young children who have poorly developed maxillary sinuses.

Clinical features

Usually presents as persistent headache and orbital cellulitis (Fig. 82) following a cold. Untreated, an orbital abscess and blindness may occur.

Management

Treatment requires hospital admission. Antibiotics are given and the maxillary sinuses washed out if also infected. Rarely, an external ethmoidectomy may be necessary. A CT scan should be performed if there is any question of an orbital abscess.

Frontal sinusitis

Potentially the most serious acute sinusitis. The long course of the frontonasal duct makes it particularly prone to obstruction by mucosal oedema.

Clinical features

Presents as frontal headache after an upper respiratory tract infection. Local tenderness is common, but may be the only sign. A sinus CT scan usually shows a fluid level or complete opacification in one or both sinuses.

Management

Treatment is with antibiotics, but sinus trephine and insertion of drainage tubes (Fig. 83) is undertaken if rapid resolution does not occur.

Sphenoiditis

Clinical features

This rare form of sinusitis may present as a deep central, retro-orbital or vertex headache. Diagnosis is confirmed by a lateral X-ray or CT scan (Fig. 84). Sinus drainage may be necessary if there is not a quick response to antibiotic therapy.

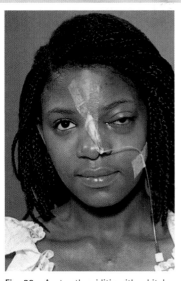

Fig. 82 Acute ethmoiditis with orbital cellulitis.

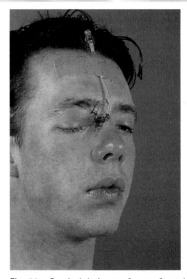

Fig. 83 Surgical drainage of acute frontal sinusitis.

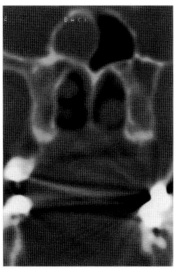

Fig. 84 Sphenoid sinus mucocele on CT scan.

Frontal sinusitis

Clinical features

Presents as a persistent frontal headache or, if a mucocele develops, a unilateral proptosis (Fig. 85). A pyocele may result from secondary infection of a mucocele. X-rays show an opaque sinus, often with hazy, indistinct edges. A CT scan will show a soft tissue mass filling the sinus (Fig. 86).

Management

Surgical treatment is aimed at re-establishing aeration of the frontal sinus. The area of the frontal recess leading into the frontal sinus can be approached either endoscopically through the nasal cavity or via an external incision. Obliteration of the frontal sinus via an osteoplastic flap approach is a radical procedure very rarely required.

Maxillary sinusitis

Aetiology

Disease is commonly bilateral unless there is an underlying septal deviation, unilateral polyp or history of maxillary trauma. A past history of dental treatment may be relevant.

Clinical features

Usually presents with chronic facial pain or upper jaw toothache. Other presentations include a purulent postnasal drip, chronic laryngitis or otitis media. Examination is often normal but paranasal sinus X-rays usually demonstrate antral disease, in the form of mucosal thickening, a persistent fluid level or total opacification.

Management

Treatment involves the creation of intranasal antrostomies to ventilate and drain the antra. Antrostomies are now normally performed endoscopically through the middle meatus. In severe cases a Caldwell–Luc approach can be used to remove diseased antral mucosa (Fig. 87).

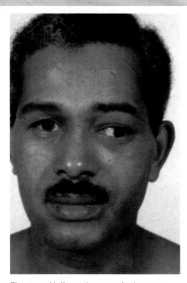

Fig. 85 Unilateral proptosis due to a mucocele.

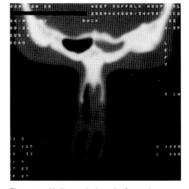

Fig. 86 Unilateral chronic frontal sinusitis.

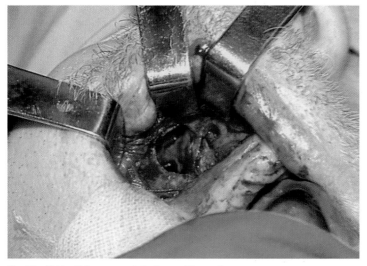

Fig. 87 Caldwell–Luc approach to the maxillary antrum.

25 › Functional endoscopic sinus surgery

The widespread availability of endoscopes and high-quality radiology has led to a reappraisal of many of the established methods of treatment for chronic sinusitis. Most sinus infections are rhinogenic, spreading from the nose into the sinuses. Both the frontal and maxillary sinuses are drained and ventilated through the narrow clefts of the anterior ethmoid cells, close to the middle nasal turbinate. It is this small area that is critical in the development of chronic sinusitis.

Diagnostic evaluation

Patients with a history suggestive of chronic sinusitis are evaluated by rigid endoscopy under local anaesthetic. The middle meatus is particularly important (Fig. 88), and is inspected for evidence of polyps, purulent secretion (Fig. 89) or anatomical abnormality that may impede sinus ventilation.

Where endoscopic surgery is necessary a CT scan in the coronal plane is obtained to show the underlying sinus anatomy (Fig. 90), the extent of chronic sinus disease (Fig. 91) and its relationship to adjacent structures such as the orbital contents and anterior cranial fossa.

Endoscopic surgery

When chronic sinusitis persists despite adequate medical treatment, patients may undergo endoscopic surgery. These operations remove diseased sinus mucosa and improve ventilation in the middle meatus area. Usually anterior ethmoidectomy is performed, but in more extensive disease access to the posterior ethmoidal and sphenoidal sinuses is possible.

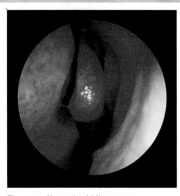

Fig. 88 Normal middle meatus.

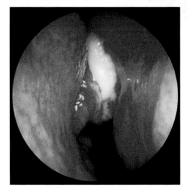

Fig. 89 Pus in the middle meatus.

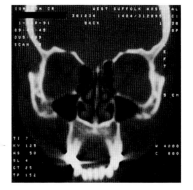

Fig. 90 Normal coronal CT scan.

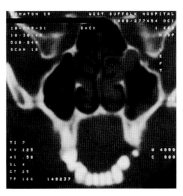

Fig. 91 CT scan with ethmoidal disease.

Lymphoid tissue found at the junction of the roof and posterior wall of the nasopharynx, thought to be involved in the development of humoral immunity as a component of the 'gut-associated lymphoid tissue' (GALT). Adenoid tissue is present at birth and during childhood, beginning to atrophy before puberty.

Clinical features

Adenoidal hypertrophy (Fig. 92) disturbs nasopharyngeal airflow and Eustachian tube function and can also act as a focus of infection for adjacent sites. Common clinical features are nasal obstruction and discharge, deafness due to middle ear effusion and otalgia due to recurrent otitis media. Gross adenoidal enlargement, often associated with tonsillar hypertrophy, can cause sleep apnoea syndrome in which apnoeic episodes during sleep are associated with daytime somnolence and in severe cases pulmonary hypertension and cor pulmonale. Clinical suspicion of enlarged adenoids can be confirmed by lateral radiography (Fig. 93).

Management

Surgical removal (adenoidectomy) can be undertaken if enlarged adenoids are causing sleep apnoea, nasal obstruction or are a contributing factor to persistent middle ear effusions or recurrent otitis media.

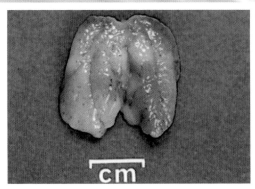

Fig. 92   Operative specimen of adenoids.

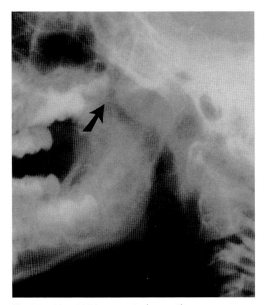

Fig. 93   Adenoidal hypertrophy (arrowed).

Nasal fractures

Clinical features

This common fracture can produce an external deformity (Fig. 94) which may be palpable, and internal disruption, e.g. septal haematoma or septal deviation. Ethmoid involvement may produce CSF rhinorrhoea.

Management

Reduce any external bony deviation under general or local anaesthesia. A septal deviation may require a submucosal resection at a later date.

Zygomatic (malar) fractures

Clinical features

Usually tripartite (Fig. 95), the cheek contour is flattened and trismus is common. Orbital movements may be limited if the orbital floor is involved.

Management

Elevation of the zygoma (via a Gillies approach) may need to be supplemented by internal wiring and antral packing, through a Caldwell–Luc approach.

Maxillary (Le Fort) fractures

There are three types of maxillary or Le Fort fracture (Fig. 96):

- Type I
- Type II
- Type III.

Clinical features

Airways obstruction by the mobile bone fragment is a serious threat. Malocclusion is common.

Management

Treatment involves fixing the mobile portion using arch bars and, frequently, bilateral suspension wiring from the frontal or parietal bones.

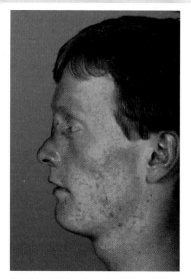

Fig. 94 Fractured nasal bones.

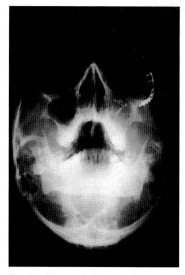

Fig. 95 Zygomatic fracture after open reduction.

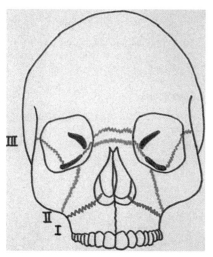

Fig. 96 Types of Le Fort maxillary fractures.

28 Tumours of the nasopharynx

Angiofibroma

Incidence

A benign vascular tumour occurring in males under the age of 25 years.

Clinical features

Nasal obstruction, epistaxis and deafness due to middle ear effusion are common characteristics.

Management

Treatment is by surgical excision, facilitated by preoperative CT scanning (Fig. 97), arteriography and embolization (Fig. 98).

Malignant tumours

Incidence

Common in south east Asia, where they account for 20% of all malignant tumours.

Clinical features

Present as nasal obstruction, epistaxis and deafness. Metastasis to cervical nodes may occur prior to local symptoms becoming apparent. Cranial nerve palsies occur in advanced cases.

Pathology

Most are squamous carcinomas, although anaplastic carcinomas and lymphomas also occur.

Management

Radiotherapy following biopsy confirmation (Fig. 99), with surgery used only for cervical nodes not responding to irradiation.

Chordoma

A very rare locally invasive neoplasm arising from remnants of the fetal notochord found in the skull base. Presents with neurological, nasal and ophthalmic symptoms.

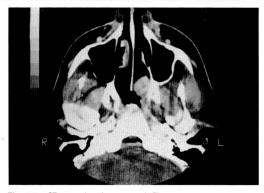

Fig. 97 CT scan showing an angiofibroma.

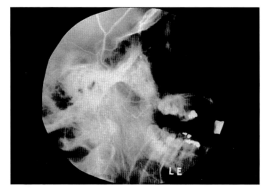

Fig. 98 Arteriogram demonstrating vascularity of angiofibroma.

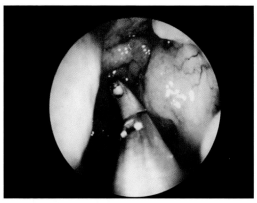

Fig. 99 Endoscopic biopsy of a nasopharyngeal carcinoma.

Pathology

Benign tumours: include papillomas, adenomas, osteomas and angiomas. The inverting papilloma may undergo malignant change.

Malignant tumours: 50% of malignant tumours are found in the maxillary sinus. Squamous cell carcinoma is the most common type. Others include adenocarcinoma, adenoid cystic carcinoma, melanoma and sarcoma.

Clinical features

Benign tumours frequently present as a unilateral nasal polyp. Malignant tumours spread medially to produce nasal obstruction or epistaxis, posteriorly to give Eustachian tube obstruction and cranial nerve palsies, inferiorly to disrupt the teeth (Fig. 100) or superiorly to give proptosis or epiphora. Lateral spread produces swelling of the cheek.

Management

Prior to treatment planning, histological diagnosis and radiological assessment of the extent of the tumour using CT scanning and sinus tomography are necessary (Fig. 101). Benign tumours are treated by local excision, either endoscopically or by an external lateral rhinotomy approach. Malignant tumours have a poor prognosis due to their late presentation and extensive spread. When curative treatment is possible a combination of radical surgery (maxillectomy) and radiotherapy is usually used. The resulting defect is filled with a dental plate and obturator (Fig. 102).

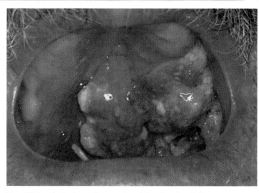

Fig. 100   Antral carcinoma involving hard palate.

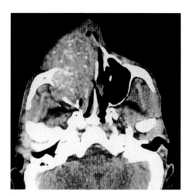

Fig. 101   Extensive antral carcinoma on CT scan.

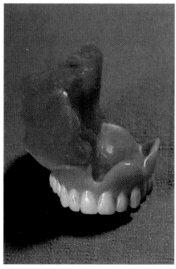

Fig. 102   Dental plate and obturator.

Nasal obstruction in children is usually noted by parents, particularly when accompanied by rhinorrhoea and snoring. Adenoid hypertrophy is the most common cause of paediatric nasal obstruction; however, the following conditions should also be borne in mind.

Posterior choanal atresia

Aetiology

A congenital condition caused by persistence of the embryonic bucconasal membrane. The obstruction is at the posterior end of the nose near the edge of the hard palate.

Clinical features

In bilateral cases there is respiratory difficulty at birth aggravated by feeding and necessitating the use of an oral airway. Unilateral cases present later with unilateral nasal obstruction and rhinorrhoea. Diagnosis is made by the inability to pass a rubber catheter through the nose into the pharynx and is confirmed by CT scanning (Fig. 103).

Management

Surgical division of the atretic plate by the transnasal or transpalatal route is required.

Nasal foreign body

A common occurrence in children, e.g. with beads, pieces of sponge or paper (Fig. 104).

Clinical features

Typically presents with unilateral foul blood-stained rhinorrhoea, nasal vestibulitis and fetor.

Management

A general anaesthetic is occasionally required for removal in an uncooperative child.

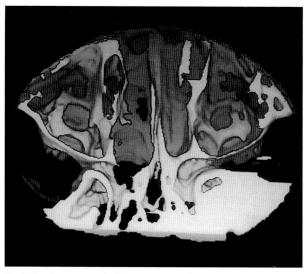

Fig. 103 Choanal atresia (3D reconstruction).

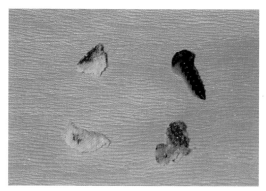

Fig. 104 Foreign bodies removed from a child's nose.

Clinical features

The hallmark of laryngeal obstruction is stridor. Inspiratory stridor indicates glottic or supraglottic obstruction, expiratory stridor bronchial obstruction and two-way stridor subglottic obstruction. If stridor is accompanied by cyanosis, tachycardia and intercostal and sternal recession (Fig. 105), urgent measures are needed to save life. In less severe cases a hoarse voice, feeding problems and recurrent chest infections may occur.

Congenital laryngeal obstruction

Aetiology

Congenital anomalies include laryngeal cysts, webs, stenosis, vascular rings and vocal cord paralysis. Laryngomalacia is a condition caused by abnormal flaccidity of the larynx allowing the supraglottic structures to be drawn into the airway on inspiration; the condition resolves with age.

Management

All cases of congenital stridor should undergo direct laryngoscopy.

Acquired laryngeal obstruction

Aetiology

Acute epiglottitis: due to *Haemophilus influenzae*. It causes rapidly progressive airway obstruction (Fig. 106).

Acute laryngotracheobronchitis (croup): due to para-influenzae virus or respiratory syncytial virus. It produces oedema, exudates and crusting of the larynx, trachea and bronchi.

Subglottic stenosis: may follow infant tracheostomy or prolonged endotracheal intubation.

Management

Acute epiglottitis: treatment is with intravenous chloramphenicol. Endotracheal intubation or an emergency tracheostomy may be necessary.

Acute laryngotracheobronchitis: endotracheal intubation is rarely required.

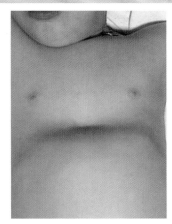

Fig. 105 Sternal recession in a child with upper airways obstruction.

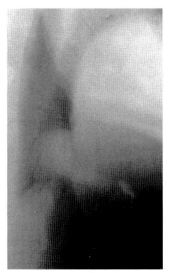

Fig. 106 Epiglottic swelling in acute epiglottitis.

32 Acute tonsillitis

Incidence	A very common disease particularly affecting children between the ages of 4 and 10 years.
Aetiology	Over 50% of the cases are due to a B haemolytic streptococcus, the majority of the others being of viral, staphylococcal or pneumococcal origin.
Clinical features	Sore throat, dysphagia, pain on swallowing and otalgia are associated with pyrexia and general malaise. The pharyngeal mucosa appears red and the tonsils are often enlarged and covered by discrete microabscesses or a confluent exudate (Fig. 107). The tonsils often remain chronically enlarged and inflamed (Fig. 108). Lymphadenopathy is frequent, the jugulo-digastric nodes being most commonly involved. A full blood count reveals a leukocytosis but a bacteriology swab does not always grow the pathogen concerned.
Differential diagnosis	*Infectious mononucleosis.* It may be impossible to distinguish between the two without a Paul–Bunnell test and a differential white cell count (the latter shows atypical monocytes and a lymphocytosis).
	Blood dyscrasias. Any white cell abnormality giving an impaired immune status may present as a severe pharyngitis, e.g. acute leukaemia.
	Diphtheria. Rarely seen but should always be borne in mind when there is a membranous exudate over the tonsils or when severe airways obstruction is evident.

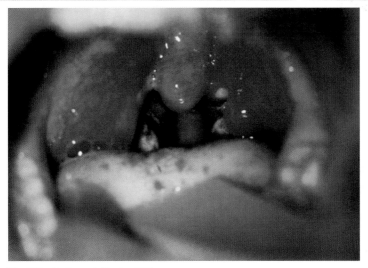

Fig. 107 Acute exudative tonsillitis.

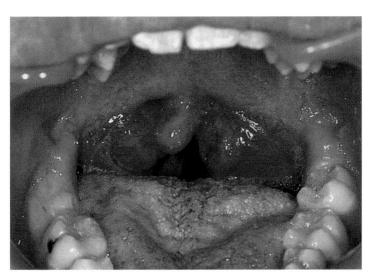

Fig. 108 Chronically enlarged tonsils following recurrent infection.

Management	Bed rest, antibiotics and adequate hydration. Penicillin is given (orally or intravenously) unless organism sensitivities or allergy dictate otherwise. In severe cases with grossly enlarged tonsils a tracheostomy may be necessary for airways obstruction.

Recurrent episodes over a prolonged period of time are best managed by tonsillectomy (Fig. 109). Following surgery the tonsillar fossae heal over a period of 7–10 days during which time they are covered by a slough (Fig. 110), which may mimic an ulcerative pharyngitis. Infection and secondary haemorrhage from the fossae can occur during this period.

Complications

- Chronic tonsillitis
- Peritonsillar abscess (quinsy) (Fig. 111): hospitalization, antibiotics and intraoral incision and drainage are required
- Parapharyngeal abscess: requires surgical drainage through an external neck incision
- Acute otitis media
- Post-streptococcal rheumatic fever/glomerulonephritis: now rare.

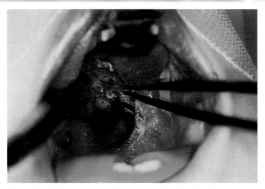

Fig. 109 Dissection tonsillectomy using bipolar diathermy.

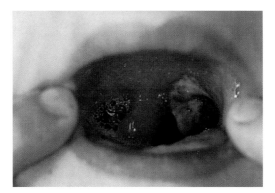

Fig. 110 Post-tonsillectomy slough overlying tonsillar fossae.

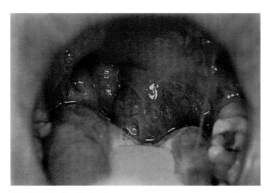

Fig. 111 Left-sided quinsy.

Acute retropharyngeal abscess

Lymphadenitis of the retropharyngeal nodes following an upper respiratory tract infection in children.

Clinical features

Presents with sore throat, pyrexia and swelling of the posterior pharyngeal wall. Lateral X-ray shows retropharyngeal swelling (Fig. 112).

Management

The abscess should be drained via the mouth with precautions taken to avoid inhalation of pus.

Chronic retropharyngeal abscess

Occurs in adults in association with tuberculous cervical spine disease.

Clinical features

Swelling is seen in the midline of the pharynx and X-rays show vertebral disease.

Management

Treatment is with antituberculous chemotherapy.

Parapharyngeal abscess

The tissue space lateral to the pharynx may become infected by spread of organisms from the tonsils or lower third molar teeth.

Clinical features

Presents with sore throat and trismus. The tonsil is pushed medially and there is neck swelling (Fig. 113).

Management

Treatment is by incision and drainage via the neck followed by appropriate antibiotic therapy.

Ludwig's angina

Clinical features

Cellulitis of the submandibular space secondary to dental disease or tonsillitis presents with swelling of the submental region (Fig. 114) and floor of the mouth.

Management

Treat with high-dose antibiotics.

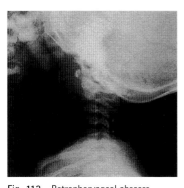

Fig. 112 Retropharyngeal abscess.

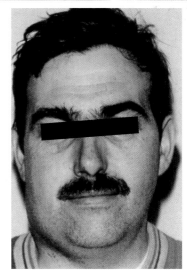

Fig. 113 Parapharyngeal abscess.

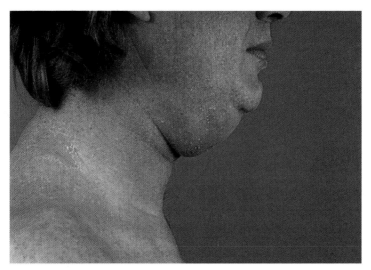

Fig. 114 Ludwig's angina.

Lingual thyroid

Aetiology

Tissue originating from the site of the foramen caecum invaginates and migrates down into the lower neck to form the thyroid gland. Thyroid tissue may be found at any point along this path of descent, e.g. lingual thyroid (Fig. 115) or thyroglossal cyst.

Clinical features

Usually presents as dysphagia. Haemorrhage and airway obstruction rarely occur.

Management

Once functioning thyroid tissue has been demonstrated elsewhere in the neck, the lump may be removed if it is causing significant symptoms.

Black hairy tongue

Aetiology

Caused by overgrowth and elongation of the filiform papillae of the anterior tongue in association with their black or brown discoloration (Fig. 116).

Clinical features

Asymptomatic, but for its appearance.

Management

Treatment is by mechanical brushing or scraping of the dorsum of the tongue.

Geographic tongue

Incidence

Affects 1% of the population.

Clinical features

Irregularly shaped areas of depapillation occur over the dorsum of the tongue (Fig. 117). The patches vary in size and distribution over a period of days.

Management

No treatment is required.

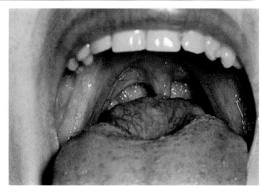

Fig. 115 Lingual thyroid.

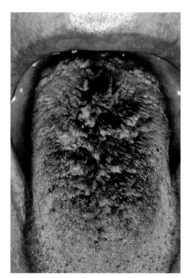

Fig. 116 Black hairy tongue.

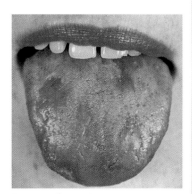

Fig. 117 Geographic tongue.

35 Leukoplakia and tongue carcinoma

Leukoplakia

A white patch which cannot be wiped away and for which no other diagnosis is apparent (Fig. 118). Risk factors in the development of oral cavity or tongue leukoplakia include alcohol, smoking, spice and betel nut chewing, syphilis and dental trauma. About 5% of cases become malignant. Exclusion of an associated carcinoma is essential.

Tongue carcinoma

Almost all tongue carcinomas are squamous in origin. There need not be any pre-existing leukoplakia.

Clinical features

May present as an exophytic or infiltrative lump on the tongue (Fig. 119). Pain and dysphagia are common. Referred otalgia (via lingual and glossopharyngeal nerves) may also occur. At presentation most tumours are greater than 2 cm diameter and 50% have palpably involved lymph nodes.

Management

Small lesions. Radiotherapy, using external beam or interstitial implant techniques (Fig. 120), or surgery, in the form of a partial or hemiglossectomy (Fig. 121) are equally effective.

Large lesions. Treatment is with radiotherapy or surgery alone or a planned combination of the two. Both modalities produce quite severe functional disability in the oral cavity, especially regarding speech and swallowing.

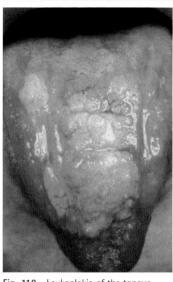

Fig. 118   Leukoplakia of the tongue.

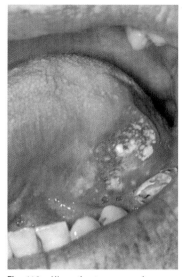

Fig. 119   Ulcerative tongue carcinoma.

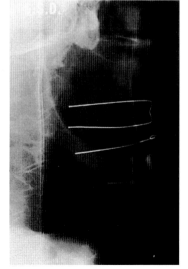

Fig. 120   Interstitial implant in the tongue.

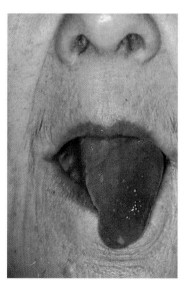

Fig. 121   Tongue after hemiglossectomy.

Benign cysts

Clinical features

Mucous retention cysts, tonsilloliths or cysts of inspissated epithelial debris may occur. They are smooth and localized to one portion of the tonsil (Fig. 122).

Management

Symptomatic cysts may be helped by tonsillectomy.

Lymphoma

Clinical features

Unilateral tonsillar swelling with an intact overlying mucosa (Fig. 123) may cause dysphagia and is suspicious of a lymphoma. The tonsil feels rubbery. Excision biopsy confirms the diagnosis.

Management

After staging the disease, treatment involves radiotherapy for localized disease, with chemotherapy being added in more advanced cases.

Carcinoma

Clinical features

Squamous carcinoma of the tonsil presents as otalgia, sore throat or dysphagia in heavy drinkers and smokers. More than 50% of cases have involved neck nodes ipsilaterally: this may be the mode of presentation. The tonsil is hard and ulcerated (Fig. 124).

Management

After full endoscopy and biopsy small primaries without nodes are best treated by radiotherapy. Surgery (which involves a block dissection of neck, partial mandibulectomy and excision of the primary) is reserved for radiation failures and large primaries.

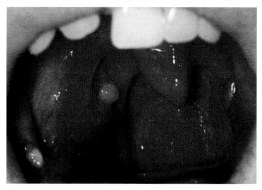

Fig. 122   Tonsil retention cyst.

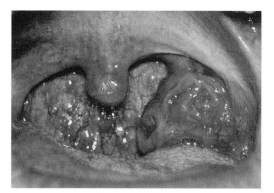

Fig. 123   Tonsil lymphoma.

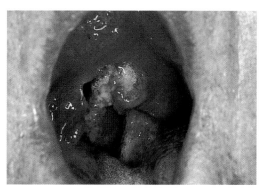

Fig. 124   Carcinoma of the right tonsil.

Diseases of the palate

Torus palatinus

Clinical features

Presents as a unilobular or multilobular bony protruberance in the midline of the hard palate (Fig. 125). The aetiology is unknown.

Management

The torus can be reduced by drilling if a denture needs to be worn or if the swelling interferes with eating.

Palatal tumours

Although these are usually due to inferior extension of a maxillary sinus tumour, benign or malignant neoplasms can arise from the palate itself (Fig. 126).

Clinical features

Presents with loose teeth, ill-fitting dentures and facial swelling. The most common types are the pleomorphic adenoma, adenoid cystic carcinoma and squamous carcinoma.

Management

Treatment is by surgical excision and/or radiotherapy, depending on the histological diagnosis.

Clefts of the palate and lip

Two of the most common congenital anomalies.

Clinical features

Clefts of the lip and palate can occur in isolation (Fig. 127) but they often occur together. Initial difficulties may be encountered with feeding, with abnormal facial development later. Palatal clefts are often associated with middle ear effusions owing to Eustachian tube dysfunction.

Management

Plastic surgical repair of clefts with long-term orthodontic care and screening for middle ear effusions.

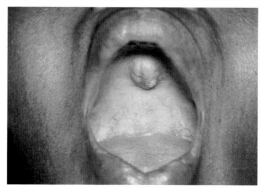

Fig. 125   Torus palatinus.

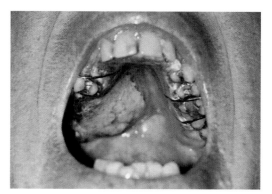

Fig. 126   Pleomorphic adenoma of the hard palate.

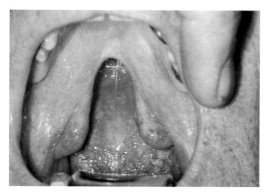

Fig. 127   Untreated cleft palate in an adult.

If symptoms of hoarseness, dysphagia, chronic sore throat or a lump in the neck continue for longer than 6 weeks, careful examination of the upper airway is mandatory. Listen to the patient's voice: is it intermittently or permanently dysphonic? The former might suggest a functional problem, the latter an organic one. A 'breathy' voice is typical of a vocal cord palsy. Also, listen for evidence of stridor. A 'hot potato' voice is indicative of supraglottic or oropharyngeal pathology.

When assessing the oral cavity and oropharynx, particular attention should be paid to mucosal ulceration or swelling. If the patient has a particularly brisk gag reflex, the palate and oropharynx should be sprayed with Lidocaine prior to attempting indirect laryngoscopy. A warmed laryngeal mirror is used to visualize the larynx while the doctor gently holds the patient's protruded tongue (Fig. 128). The patient should mouth breathe. Vocal cord movement is assessed by asking the patient to say 'Hey!' If the technique is not tolerated, then the patient's better nasal airway is locally anaesthetized and a fibre-optic scope is used to examine the larynx and pharynx (Fig. 129).

Both the nose and neck should be routinely examined as part of the assessment of the upper airway.

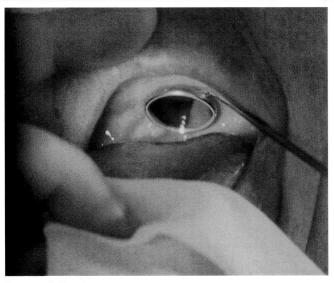

Fig. 128 Indirect laryngoscopy.

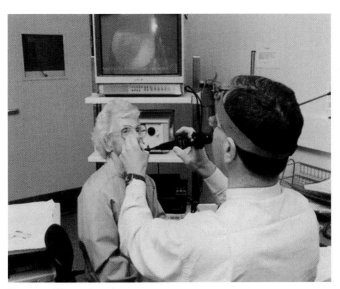

Fig. 129 Fibre-optic endoscopy.

Chronic non-specific laryngitis

Aetiology

Common. Usually associated with vocal abuse, smoking or sepsis elsewhere in the respiratory tract, e.g. chronic sinusitis.

Clinical features

Hoarseness may be accompanied by sore throat. Indirect laryngoscopy may distinguish localized forms, e.g. singer's nodules (Fig. 130), Reinke's oedema (Fig. 131) or laryngeal polyps, from the generalized forms, e.g. chronic hypertrophic laryngitis (Fig. 132).

Management

Treatment involves the removal of any precipitating factors and speech therapy is important. Localized polyps or nodules may merit endoscopic removal.

Chronic specific laryngitis

Rare. Most of the granulomatous diseases can involve the larynx, e.g. tuberculosis, syphilis, sarcoidosis, scleroma or Wegener's granulomatosis.

Management

The lesions may mimic a carcinoma and a direct laryngoscopy and biopsy is mandatory. Treatment is that of the underlying systemic condition.

Leukoplakia

Usually affects the true cords (Fig. 133). The aetiology is as for chronic non-specific laryngitis. Microscopically, the findings of hyperkeratosis and dysplasia are common, although in situ or invasive carcinoma can only be excluded by an adequate biopsy.

Management

Endoscopy should be undertaken in all cases. Leukoplakia should be regarded as having the potential to undergo malignant change.

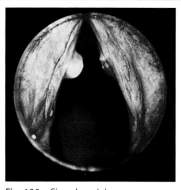

Fig. 130   Singer's nodules.

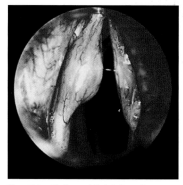

Fig. 131   Unilateral Reinke's oedema.

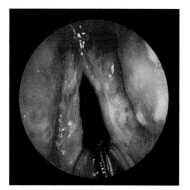

Fig. 132   Chronic hypertrophic laryngitis.

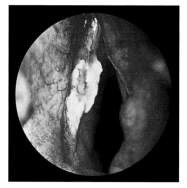

Fig. 133   Leukoplakia of the left true vocal cord.

Papilloma

Aetiology

Localized infection with human papillomavirus (HPV).

Clinical features

In the child (juvenile form): multiple lesions that may spread to the trachea and bronchi. Cases may regress at puberty.

In the adult: less common and usually a single lesion.

Both forms present with hoarseness or airway obstruction.

Management

Endoscopic removal (Fig. 134) using either suction diathermy or a CO_2 laser. Surgical seeding of lesions within the larynx or trachea is common, and removal may be necessary for frequent recurrence.

Carcinoma

Aetiology

Associated with cigarette smoking and high alcohol intake, although the latter is more important in causing piriform fossa carcinoma.

Clinical features

Usually presents as persistent hoarseness. Dysphagia, chronic cough, stridor and referred otalgia may also occur. Occasionally a supraglottic tumour may present with metastatic neck nodes. The tumour may be evident on indirect laryngoscopy but endoscopic assessment (Fig. 135) and biopsy are mandatory before deciding on the appropriate treatment. A second primary (1%) in the upper aerodigestive tract should be searched for at this time. Fine-needle aspiration cytology of any suspicious neck mass should also be undertaken. A CT scan will show any spread outside the larynx, or involvement of laryngeal cartilages.

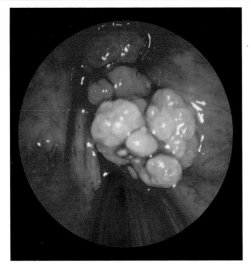

Fig. 134 Endoscopic appearance of laryngeal papillomata.

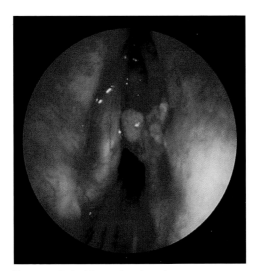

Fig. 135 Early right vocal cord carcinoma.

Management

Small (T1 and T2) carcinomas are best treated with primary radiotherapy, laryngectomy being reserved for post-radiation recurrences, larger (T3 and T4) lesions (Fig. 136) and primary tumours associated with neck nodes greater than 2 cm in diameter. Primary endoscopic excision of laryngeal carcinomas with a carbon dioxide laser is now being undertaken by some surgeons.

Voice rehabilitation

Following total laryngectomy the patient may be able to speak again by:

- learning oesophageal speech (swallowed air is voluntarily regurgitated through the pharynx)
- using an artificial larynx (Fig. 138), which transmits vibrations into the pharynx and oral cavity while the patient articulates
- surgical provision of a tracheo-oesophageal fistula, which is fitted with a button or valve (Fig. 137). The button has a one-way flutter valve, which allows airflow from the trachea into the pharynx when the tracheostome is occluded. In selected patients this enables the development of good voice.

Results

Patients require close follow-up. Recurrences can develop in the larynx, pharynx, stoma or neck. Further surgery or radiotherapy may be indicated. The expected 5-year survival for a T1 laryngeal cancer is about 95%. This falls to about 50% for T4 disease.

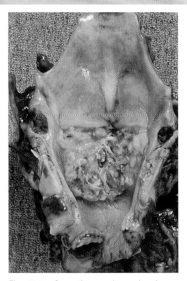

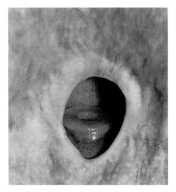

Fig. 136 Operative specimen showing extensive laryngeal carcinoma.

Fig. 137 Blom–Singer valve in situ.

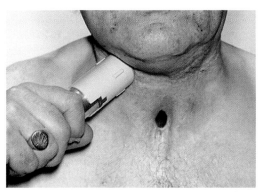

Fig. 138 Patient using an 'artificial larynx'.

Oropharynx

Fish bones may lodge in the tonsil or tongue base.

Clinical features

The patient complains of pain on swallowing and points to the suprahyoid region. The bone may only be obvious on palpation: X-rays are unhelpful.

Management

Removal under direct vision.

Hypopharynx/oesophagus

A bone or food bolus usually gets lodged at one of four sites:

- one piriform fossa
- the postcricoid region (15 cm from the upper incisor)
- the level of the aortic arch (at 25 cm)
- at the oesophago-gastric junction (40 cm).

Clinical features

Dysphagia may be total, the patient spitting out saliva and pointing to the suprasternal or retrosternal region. A soft tissue lateral X-ray of the neck may delineate a bone (Fig. 139).

Management

Endoscopic removal should be undertaken as soon as possible, to avoid airway oedema, soft tissue infection or oesophageal perforation.

Bronchus

Often a peanut in a young child.

Clinical features

After an initial coughing fit there is often a latent period before respiratory distress becomes obvious. The chest X-ray may show collapse of the lung distally, if the obstruction is complete, or emphysema of the involved side if the obstruction acts as a one-way valve (Fig. 140).

Management

Bronchoscopic removal is mandatory.

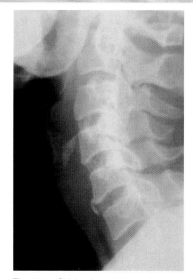

Fig. 139 Chicken bone in hypopharynx.

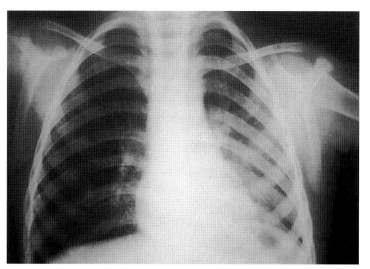

Fig. 140 Peanut in right main bronchus, demonstrating ipsilateral emphysema.

Thyroglossal cyst

Most common midline neck cyst (Fig. 141) usually presenting in childhood.

Clinical features

Painless, unless infected, and moves on protrusion of tongue. Sinus formation may follow previous infection or incomplete excision.

Management

If a thyroid scan shows functioning tissue elsewhere, then excise with central portion of hyoid bone and tract up to foramen caecum (Sistrunk's operation).

Branchial cyst and fistula

Aetiology

Represent branchial apparatus remnants. The fistula results from persistence of the second pouch and cervical sinus.

Clinical features

Cysts usually lie deep to the anterior border of sternomastoid, presenting with a painless neck swelling or mimicking a parapharyngeal abscess if infection occurs. A complete branchial fistula has its internal opening in the region of the tonsil and an external opening anterior to sternomastoid. Diagnosis can be confirmed by needle aspiration of cyst contents.

Management

Excision, with any fistulous tract.

Cystic hygroma

A variety of lymphangioma.

Clinical features

A soft, transilluminable mass usually presenting in the parotid region in the first year of life (Fig. 142).

Management

Excision, which may have to be incomplete because of the diffuse infiltration of soft tissues by the tumour.

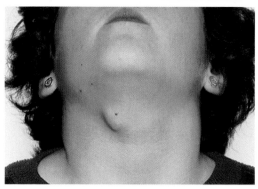

Fig. 141   Thyroglossal cyst.

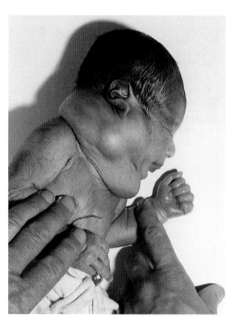

Fig. 142   Cystic hygroma of the right parotid gland.

A tracheostomy is an artificial opening made into the trachea. It may be created after the larynx has been removed, when it is permanent, or when the larynx is still in place, when it is usually temporary (Fig. 143).

Indications

- Total laryngectomy
- Airway protection, e.g. after major head and neck surgery, neurological disease involving the larynx
- Airway obstruction, e.g. epiglottitis, bilateral recurrent laryngeal nerve palsy, tumour
- Respiratory insufficiency (when endotracheal intubation required for longer than 72 h), e.g. severe chest wall injury, Guillain–Barré syndrome.

Surgical technique

- Incision. Horizontal, midway between the cricoid cartilage and suprasternal notch.
- Vertical incision and separation of strap muscles.
- Transfixion and separation of thyroid isthmus.
- Creation of an opening into the trachea. In adults a window is cut out (Fig. 144). A vertical slit incision is used in children. A trap-door flap should not be used.
- Insertion of tracheostomy tube. A correctly sized cuffed synthetic tube is used for the first 24 h. This can be replaced later on by an uncuffed tube (Fig. 145).

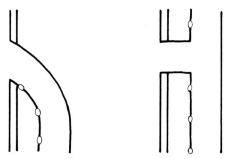

Fig. 143 Types of tracheostomy.

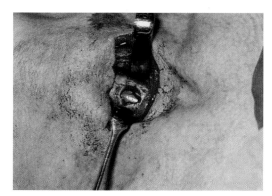

Fig. 144 Window cut in anterior tracheal wall.

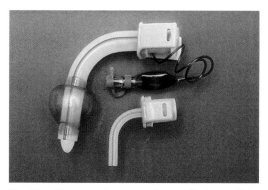

Fig. 145 Silicone tracheostomy tubes: paediatric uncuffed and adult cuffed.

| Complications | *Immediate.* Pneumothorax, haemorrhage, surgical emphysema and tube displacement can all occur. |

Early. Wound infection, dysphagia and tube obstruction are all common. Tracheal erosion with innominate artery rupture, perichondritis and apnoea in hypercapnoeic bronchitics are rare.

Late. Tracheal stenosis may result from prolonged or overinflation of the cuffed tube. Decannulation may be difficult in children. Surgical closure of a persistent tracheocutaneous fistula is rarely required after decannulation.

Stomal stenosis

Aetiology

Following laryngectomy the lower end of the trachea is brought out through the neck skin. Local wound infection, radiotherapy and keloid formation all predispose to the later development of a stomal stenosis (Fig. 146). The other cause of stomal stenosis is recurrence of tumour (Fig. 147).

Management

Management of benign stomal stenosis is either by the permanent wearing of a stoma button or laryngectomy tube or by surgical revision of the stoma.

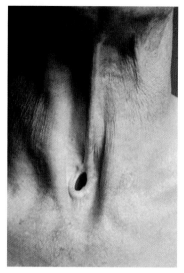

Fig. 146   Stomal stenosis due to scar tissue.

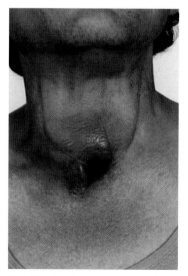

Fig. 147   Post-laryngectomy stomal recurrence.

Pharyngeal pouch

Aetiology

A pharyngeal pouch develops from a herniation of pharyngeal mucosa through Killian's dehiscence.

Clinical features

Dysphagia and regurgitation of food occur. Large pouches may cause aspiration pneumonia. Pooling of saliva in the hypopharynx may be noted on indirect laryngoscopy. Barium swallow confirms the diagnosis (Fig. 148).

Management

Following an endoscopy to exclude an associated carcinoma, the pouch may be excised via an external approach or the wall between the pouch and oesophagus divided endoscopically using a stapling gun (Fig. 149).

Laryngocele

Aetiology

Distension of the laryngeal saccule can produce an internal or external laryngocele (Fig. 150).

Clinical features

Hoarseness or dysphagia may occur. External laryngoceles may produce a swelling in the neck accentuated by performing Valsalva's manoeuvre. Laryngeal tomograms taken during this manoeuvre will demonstrate the laryngocele (Fig. 151).

Management

Following endoscopy to exclude an associated carcinoma, an internal laryngocele can be 'uncapped' whilst an external laryngocele is excised through the neck.

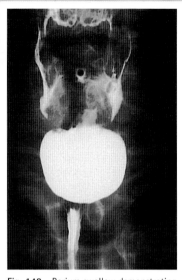

Fig. 148 Barium swallow demonstrating a pharyngeal pouch.

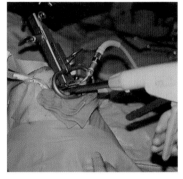

Fig. 149 The use of an endoscopic stapling gun for the treatment of a pharyngeal pouch.

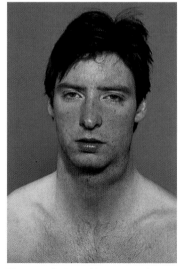

Fig. 150 Patient with an external laryngocele.

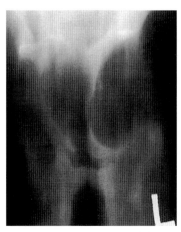

Fig. 151 Tomogram outlining air-filled laryngocele.

45 Diseases of the floor of the mouth

Anatomy

Formed largely by the anterior two-thirds of the tongue and by reflection of mucosa from the sides of the tongue to the gum on the mandible. In the midline the lingual frenulum separates the orifices of the left and right submandibular ducts. Under the mucosa lie the sublingual salivary glands.

Ranula

Aetiology

A cystic lesion arising from the sublingual gland. Usually presents in the floor of the mouth as a bluish, fluctuant swelling (Fig. 152). Less commonly the 'plunging ranula' can present as a lump in the neck.

Treatment

For lesions confined to the floor of the mouth, marsupialization is usually adequate, although recurrence can occur. Plunging ranulae require formal excision via an external neck approach.

Squamous carcinoma

Clinical features

An ulcer in the floor of the mouth which may be painful with referred otalgia (Fig. 153). Early spread to cervical nodes, which may be bilateral, is common.

Treatment

Excision of the tumour with plastic surgical reconstruction and adjuvant radiotherapy.

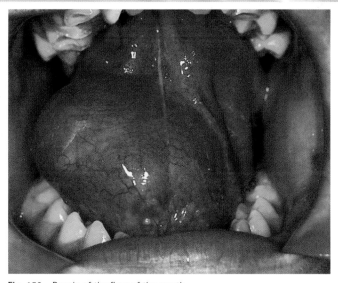

Fig. 152 Ranula of the floor of the mouth.

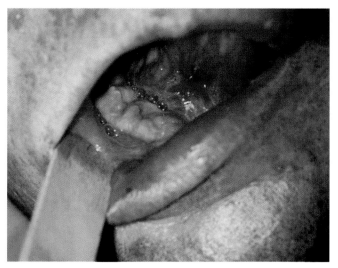

Fig. 153 Carcinoma of the floor of the mouth.

46 > Diseases of the submandibular gland

The superficial portion of the gland lies on the mylohyoid muscle; the deep portion extends around the posterior edge of muscle into the floor of the mouth. Wharton's duct leaves the deep part of the gland and runs forward to open into the anterior floor of the mouth, just lateral to the midline.

Swelling of the gland may be due to inflammation or tumour (Fig. 154).

Inflammatory disease

Clinical features

A tense, tender swelling usually results from a stone in the duct. This may be palpable bi-manually or evident on X-ray (Fig. 155). There are several lymph nodes in the submandibular triangle and enlargement of these may mimic disease in the gland.

Management

Treatment is with antibiotics and excision of the stone perorally. If this cannot be achieved, the whole gland may need to be removed by an external approach. Established infection may proceed to abscess formation.

Tumours

Fine-needle aspiration of the mass should be performed. About 50% of tumours are benign, most commonly pleomorphic adenomas.

Management

These should be excised with the entire gland, taking care to preserve the marginal mandibular branch of the facial nerve. Malignant tumours necessitate excision of the whole gland, with a radical neck dissection in certain cases.

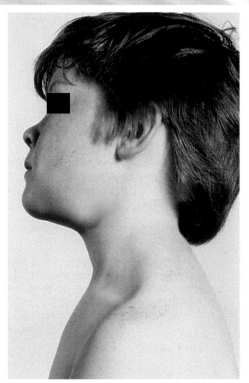

Fig. 154 Enlargement of the submandibular gland due to chronic infection.

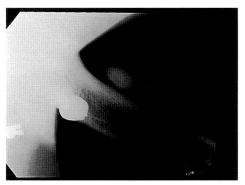

Fig. 155 Floor of mouth X-ray demonstrating a stone in the submandibular gland duct.

Mumps

Clinical features

Usually seen in children, this is the most common cause of bilateral parotid gland swelling (Fig. 156). The glands are painful and tender.

Management

Treatment is supportive, the adenopathy subsiding over a period of several days.

Acute parotid abscess

Usually seen in association with poor oral hygiene, with or without dental caries.

Clinical features

The gland becomes acutely tender with obvious inflammation of the soft tissues (Fig. 157). A stone may be palpable in the duct or evident on plain X-ray.

Management

Treatment with antibiotics should be followed by drainage via a parotidectomy approach if the swelling becomes fluctuant.

Parotid gland tumours

Types

Benign: e.g. pleomorphic adenoma (Fig. 158), Warthin's tumour

Malignant: e.g. adenoid cystic, squamous cell or adenocarcinoma, lymphoma

Clinical features

Usually painless, the speed of growth reflects the likelihood of malignancy. A facial palsy indicates a malignant tumour. Fine-needle aspiration of the mass may facilitate preoperative diagnosis.

Management

Superficial parotidectomy should be undertaken when indicated. Malignant tumours may require a total parotidectomy with sacrifice of the facial nerve.

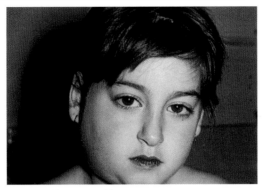

Fig. 156 Mumps parotitis.

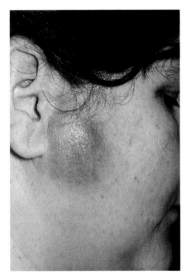

Fig. 157 Acute parotid abscess.

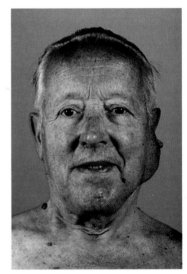

Fig. 158 Pleomorphic adenoma of the parotid gland.

Following excision of a tumour from the head or neck, primary closure of a resultant tissue defect with preservation of adequate function may not be feasible or cosmetically acceptable. Only by the introduction of tissue from another site can a satisfactory result be achieved. Such tissue may be used to provide lining (reconstruction of an internal mucosal defect) or cover (reconstruction of a skin defect).

Techniques

Non-vascularized free grafts. These depend on the recipient site for their blood supply: include split skin, full-thickness skin, dermis, nerve and bone grafts.

Pedicled skin. May be random, with a non-specific blood supply, or axial, when the flap has a named arterial blood supply, e.g. deltopectoral flap (Fig. 159) and pectoralis major myocutaneous flap (Fig. 160).

Revascularized free grafts. The artery and vein supplying the graft tissue are re-anastomosed to vessels at the recipient site. Include radial forearm flap (Fig. 161) and jejunum.

Pedicled viscera. Stomach or colon may be used.

Several factors will determine the choice of flap/ graft for the individual patient.

Myocutaneous flaps and revascularized free grafts have meant that the lining of an internal surface can be carried out as a one-stage procedure, greatly reducing hospitalization time.

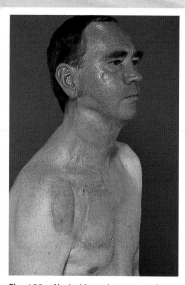

Fig. 159 Neck skin replacement using a deltopectoral flap.

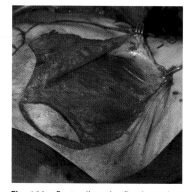

Fig. 160 Pectoralis major flap just prior to division of the muscles' attachments.

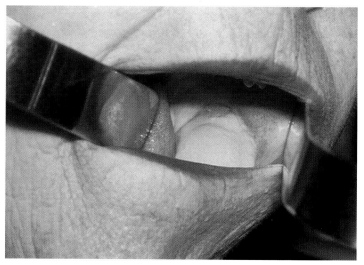

Fig. 161 Intra-orally placed radial free flap.

49 > Palsies of the last four cranial nerves

Aetiology	Often involved with lesions in the brainstem or at the skull base, e.g. with CVA, motor neurone disease, glomus tumour, meningitis and nasopharyngeal carcinoma.

Glossopharyngeal nerve

This nerve is sensory to the posterior third of the tongue (including taste) and pharyngeal mucosa. Motor to middle constrictor.

Clinical features	It is rarely paralysed alone. A unilateral palsy does not produce severe functional disability.

Vagus nerve

This nerve is sensory to the larynx and motor to the soft palate, pharynx and larynx. Also sensorimotor to the thoraco-abdominal viscera.

Aetiology	An isolated palsy of the recurrent laryngeal branch is usually either idiopathic or due to disruption of the nerve in the neck or chest, e.g. post-thyroidectomy and bronchial carcinoma (Fig. 162).
Clinical features	Variable. Palatal paralysis, hoarseness, weak cough, overspill of food and secretions and airways obstruction may all occur, although a recurrent laryngeal nerve palsy will not produce palatal paralysis.
Management	Airway incompetence due to a unilateral cord palsy may be helped by injection of Teflon into the para-cordal tissues to increase the cord's bulk or a thyroplasty could be performed (Fig. 163). Bilateral palsies may produce total airway obstruction or serious overspill. A tracheostomy will be required in either case.

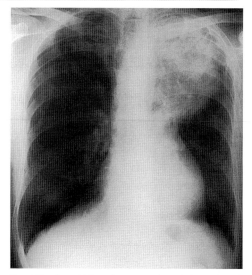

Fig. 162   Bronchial carcinoma causing a left vocal cord palsy.

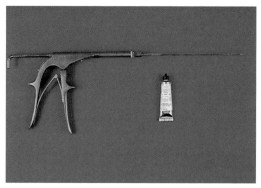

Fig. 163   Teflon gun for endoscopic injection of a paralysed vocal cord.

Accessory nerve

The spinal part of this nerve is motor to sternomastoid and trapezius. An isolated palsy is seen after a block dissection of neck or injudicious posterior triangle lymph node biopsy.

Clinical features

The shoulder assumes a dropped appearance (Fig. 164) and the patient is unable to shrug or abduct the shoulder to a vertical position.

Management

A resultant frozen shoulder may benefit from physiotherapy.

Hypoglossal nerve

This nerve is motor to tongue and hyoid depressors. An isolated palsy is usually iatrogenic, e.g. following laryngectomy or submandibular gland excision, or due to malignant disease in the upper neck.

Clinical features

On protrusion the tongue deviates to the paralysed side (Fig. 165). Wasting and fasciculation indicate lower motor neurone damage. Unilateral palsies are usually asymptomatic. Bilateral palsies produce severe dysarthria and swallowing difficulties.

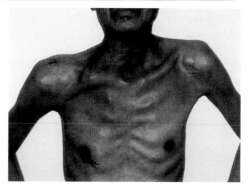

Fig. 164 Dropped shoulder following right neck dissection (and laryngectomy).

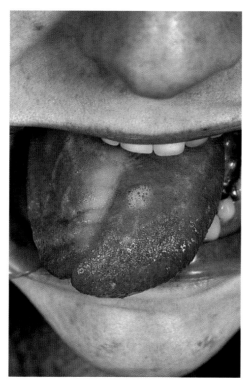

Fig. 165 Hypoglossal nerve palsy with deviation and wasting of hemitongue.

Human immunodeficiency virus (HIV) infection

ENT manifestations of HIV infection commonly fall into one of three groups.

Cervical lymphadenopathy

Clinical features

Common. May be persistent generalized lymphadenopathy (PGL) or secondary to pharyngitis. However, rapidly enlarging, asymmetrical (Fig. 166) or fixed nodes may herald a lymphoma, Kaposi's sarcoma or an occult squamous carcinoma.

Management

In cases where malignancy requires exclusion, fine-needle or open biopsy is necessary. The treatment will then depend on the pathological diagnosis.

Kaposi's sarcoma (KS)

The skin and mucosa of the head and neck are common sites for KS in AIDS patients.

Clinical features

Lesions present as red or purple macules, plaques or nodules. Palatal involvement is most common (Fig. 167). Rarely, KS may cause airway obstruction.

Management

Treatment is multi-modal.

Oral cavity 'hairy' leukoplakia

Clinical features

Leukoplakic patches on the lateral border and ventral surface of the tongue (Fig. 168) that have a tendency to regress and recur. Possibly caused by the Epstein–Barr virus (EBV). Microscopically the keratin whorls give a hairy appearance. The lesion should be distinguished from candidiasis, also common in these patients. Rapid progression to full blown AIDS is common once 'hairy' leukoplakia has developed.

Management

Treatment is by biopsy and observation of the lesion, the malignant potential of which remains unknown.

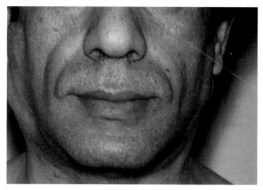

Fig. 166　Asymmetrical cervical lymphadenopathy in PGL.

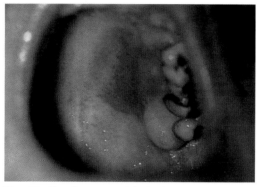

Fig. 167　Kaposi's sarcoma of the hard palate.

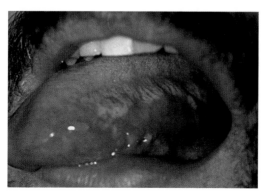

Fig. 168　Hairy leukoplakia of the lateral border of the tongue.

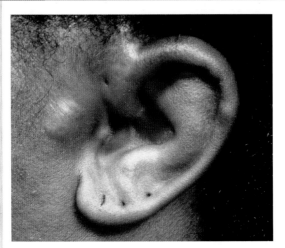

1. This 24-year-old lady has four small holes in her left pinna. Recently the anterior hole has become swollen and painful.

a. What is the nature of the holes?
b. How should her recent symptoms be managed?

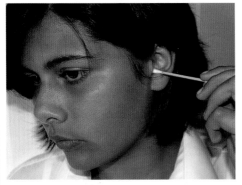

2. This photograph shows a patient 'cleaning' her ear with a cotton-tipped applicator.

a. Is this a good way to remove wax from the ear?
b. Does wax have to be removed from the ear? If not, why not?
c. What are the dangers of using cotton-tipped applicators in the ear?

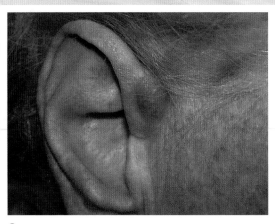

3. This photograph shows a lesion near the right pinna of a 72-year-old woman. The lesion has previously become red and swollen, with discharge of purulent material.

a. What is the most likely diagnosis?
b. What is the most appropriate treatment?

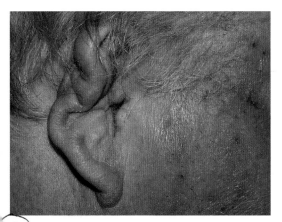

4. This 54-year-old man presented to hospital with a facial rash. He used to play rugby football when younger. Recently he has had irritation in his right ear.

a. Describe the appearance of the right ear and the likely pathology.
b. What is the rash caused by?
c. What is the treatment?

5. This 11-year-old girl presented to an ENT clinic with unilateral conductive deafness.

a. What is the diagnosis?
b. What is the treatment?

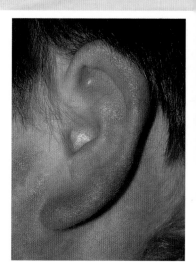

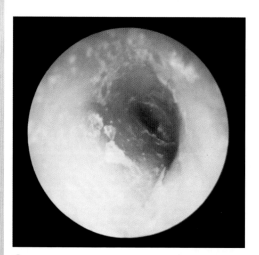

6. This is the otoscopic appearance of the right ear in a 38-year-old man who has suffered for many years with intermittent aural discharge. Recently he has noticed some difficulty with hearing.

a. Describe the otoscopic appearance.
b. How does this condition arise?
c. What is the treatment?

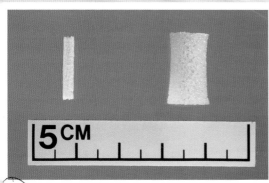

7. This photograph shows a dressing used in the treatment of ear disease.

a. What ear condition is the dressing primarily used for?
b. What is the principle behind the use of this dressing?

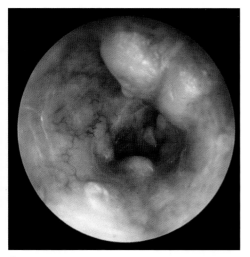

8. This is the otoscopic appearance of the right ear in a 29-year-old man who suffers with recurrent episodes of pain and discharge from the ear.

a. What is the diagnosis?
b. What activities predispose to the development of this condition?
c. What is the treatment?

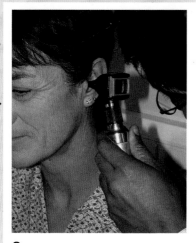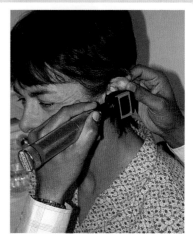

9. These photographs show two ways of examining the ear with an otoscope.

a. Which is the correct method of examination and why?

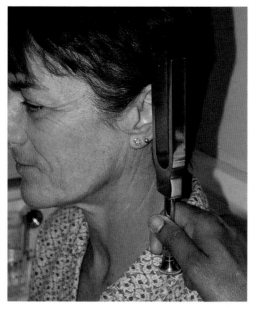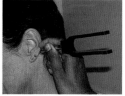

10. These photographs show a tuning fork being used to assess hearing.

a. What is the name of this particular test?
b. How does this test distinguish between different types of deafness?
c. What is the frequency of the tuning fork usually used and why?

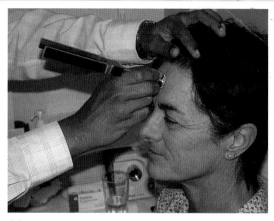

11. This photograph also shows a tuning fork assessment of hearing.

a. What is the name of this test?
b. How does this distinguish between different types of deafness?

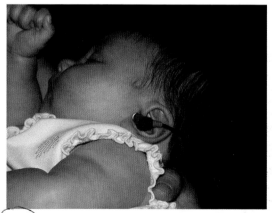

12. This photograph shows a baby undergoing an investigation in the neonatal period.

a. What is the name of the investigation?
b. What is the investigation designed to establish and why is this important?

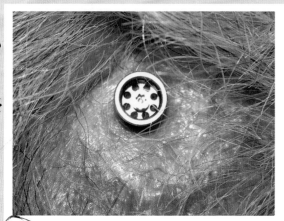

13. This photograph shows the healed operation site of a 48–year–old man with bilateral conductive deafness.   BAHA

a. What operation has been performed?
b. Why has this operation been necessary?

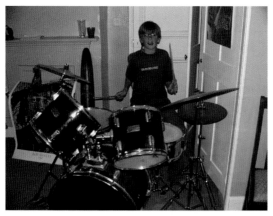

14. This teenager is indulging in a hobby.

a. What is the principle health hazard of this pastime?
b. What are the likely symptoms?
c. What is the treatment?

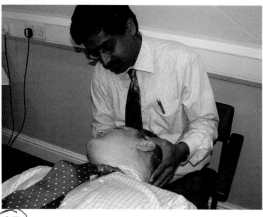

Eply particle repositioning manoeuvre
BPPV
benign paroxysmal positional vertigo

15. This photograph shows a manoeuvre used to treat a disorder of balance.

a. What is the name of this manoeuvre and what condition is being treated?
b. What is the rationale behind this treatment?

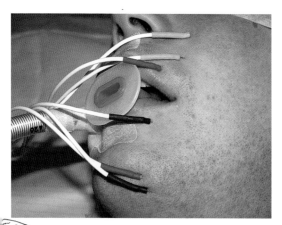

16. This photograph shows a form of intraoperative monitoring during head and neck surgery.

a. What physiological function is being monitored? *facial n. fx*
b. During what operations would this equipment be used?
c. What precautions would the anaesthetist need to take?

17. This patient has had an operation on his right ear for cholesteatoma and finds it difficult to wear a normal conventional hearing aid.

a. What operation was performed for cholesteatoma and why does this make conventional hearing aid use difficult?
b. What type of hearing aid is the patient using?

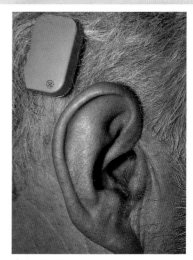

Nasopharyngeal carcinoma
(Chinese origin)
EBV.

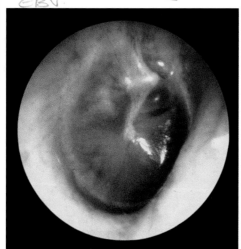

18. This is the otoscopic appearance of a 65-year-old woman who presents with deafness. She also presents with a mass of lymph nodes on the right side of the neck.

a. What is the diagnosis?
b. What is the most likely underlying pathology?
c. In which racial group is this condition most common?
d. What is the management?

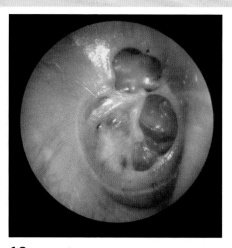

19. This is the otoscopic appearance of the right ear of a 17-year-old boy who has had hearing problems for many years.

a. Describe the otoscopic features.
b. What type of treatment is he likely to have had in the past?
c. What is the current management?

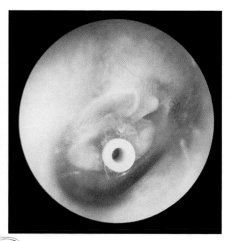

20. This is the otoscopic appearance of the right ear of a 6-year-old boy who 6 months earlier underwent an operation on both ears.

a. What operation took place?
b. What was the underlying condition for which surgery was necessary?
c. What alternative methods of treatment exist for this condition?
d. Would it be advisable for the child to swim?

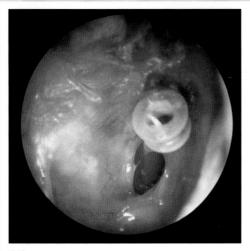

21. This is the otoscopic appearance of the right tympanic membrane in a 5-year-old girl.

a. Describe the otoscopic features.
b. What is the likely course of events during the following three months?

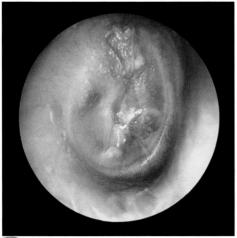

granular
myringitis

22. This is the otoscopic appearance of the right tympanic membrane of a 23-year-old man.

a. What is the diagnosis?
b. What are the symptoms?
c. What is the treatment?

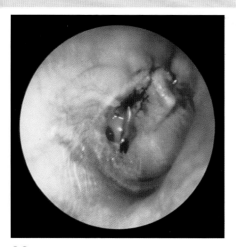

23. This is the otoscopic appearance of the right ear in a 23-year-old man who complained of deafness following a blow to the side of the head in a soccer match.

a. What is the diagnosis?
b. How is this managed?

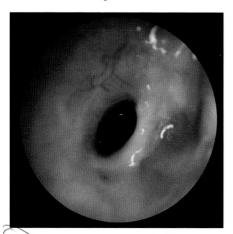

24. This is the otoscopic appearance of the right tympanic membrane of a man who has returned from a scuba diving holiday. During one dive he experienced a sharp pain in his ear. Over the following days he developed a purulent discharge from the ear.

a. What is the diagnosis?
b. What are the microbial organisms most likely to be involved?
c. How is this managed?

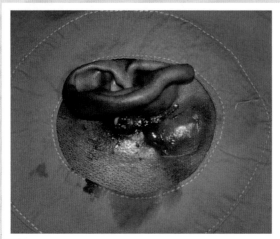

25. This is the ear of an 11-year-old Nepali girl presenting with a 2-year history of ear symptoms.

a. What does the photograph show?
b. What is the most likely underlying pathology?

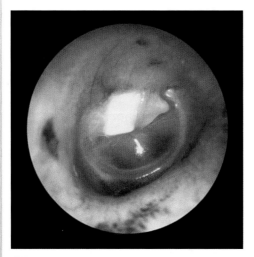

26. This is the otoscopic appearance of the right ear in a 32-year-old man who has undergone middle ear surgery.

a. Describe the otoscopic appearance
b. What operation has the patient undergone?

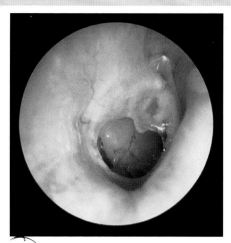

27. This is the otoscopic appearance of the right ear in an 18-year-old woman.

a. What is the diagnosis?
b. What type of deafness is usually seen in this condition?
c. What factors determine the degree of deafness?

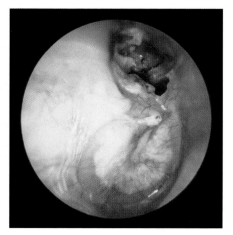

28. This is the otoscopic appearance of the right ear in a 25-year-old man who complained of recurrent discharge from the ear.

a. What is the diagnosis?
b. What are the possible complications of this condition?
c. What is the treatment?

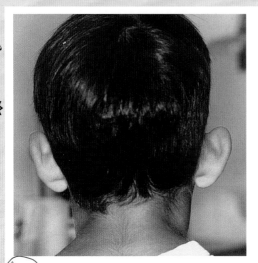

29. This photograph shows the back of a 9-year-old boy's head. Look at the appearance of the external ears.

a. Describe the appearance of the ears.
b. What is the differential diagnosis?
c. What measures would you take to confirm the diagnosis?

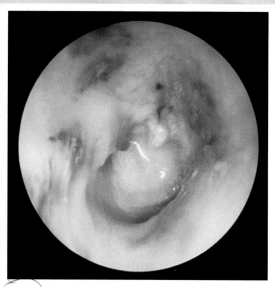

30. This is the otoscopic appearance of the right ear in a 17-year-old boy who presented with painful red swelling behind the ear. He had a history of discharge from the ear and had undergone grommet insertion on three occasions between the ages of 4 and 11 years.

a. Describe the otoscopic appearance; what is the diagnosis of the middle ear pathology?
b. What complication has arisen?
c. What is the treatment of the complication and the underlying ear disease?

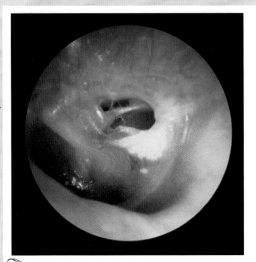

31. This is the otoscopic appearance of the left ear in a 42–year–old man with mild deafness and occasional discharge from the ear.

a. What is the diagnosis?
b. What parts of the middle ear ossicular chain are visible?

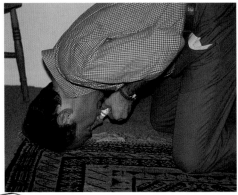

32. This middle–aged man is self–administering nasal medication.

a. What is the likely nature of the medication?
b. Why is the patient adopting this position?
c. What conditions are treated in this way?
d. What are the dangers of this medication?

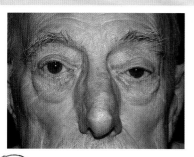 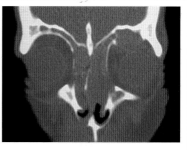

33. This photograph shows an 82-year-old man with a recent onset of double vision (diplopia). His corresponding sinus CT scan is also shown.

a. Describe the clinical appearance.
b. What dose the sinus CT show and how has the sinus pathology caused the diplopia?

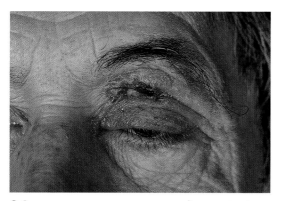

34. This photograph shows a 54-year-old man with a discharging lesion above the left eye. He also complains of nasal stuffiness and purulent nasal discharge, present for 3 months.

a. How might the discharging lesion be related to the nasal symptoms?
b. How should this case be managed?

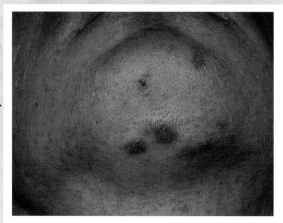

35. This photograph shows lesions on the facial skin in a 44-year-old man who has positive antibodies for human immunodeficiency virus (HIV).

a. What is the diagnosis of the facial lesions?
b. What is the treatment of the facial lesions?

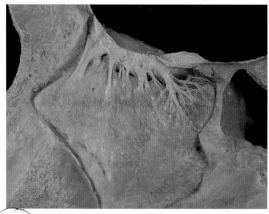

36. This cadaver section shows the nasal septum.

a. What anatomical structures form the nasal septum?
b. What are the filamentous structures at the top of the septum and what is their function?

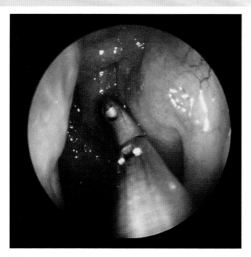

37. This is an endoscopic view of a biopsy being taken from the nasopharynx in a 54-year-old male presenting with a lump in the neck and unilateral deafness.

a. What pathology is suspected in the nasopharynx and what population group is particularly likely to suffer from this condition?
b. Explain the lump in the neck and unilateral deafness.

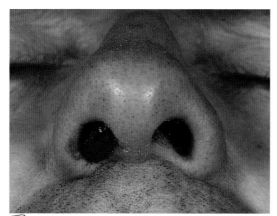

38. This photograph shows the nose of a 67-year-old man.

a. Describe the appearance.
b. What is the differential diagnosis?
c. What symptoms would suggest serious pathology?

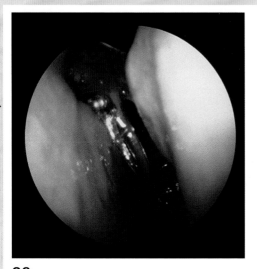

39. This photograph shows the endoscopic appearance of the nasal cavity in a patient complaining of 'catarrh'.

a. Describe the endoscopic appearance, and the nature of 'catarrh'.
b. What can be done about this symptom?

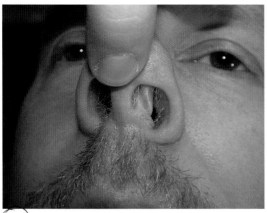

40. This photograph shows the nose of a patient with nasal blockage.

a. What is the cause of the nasal blockage?
b. What treatment would be possible?

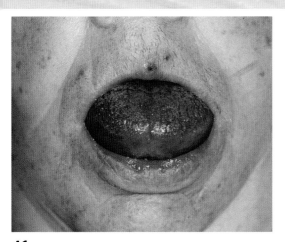

41. This photograph shows the tongue of a 63-year-old lady who presented to an accident and emergency department with an acute onset of tongue swelling.

a. What is the differential diagnosis?
b. What airway support would be appropriate?
c. What drugs might be used in the acute treatment?

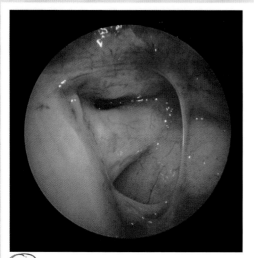

42. This is the endoscopic view of a structure seen in the sphenoid sinus during endoscopic sinus surgery, damage to which would result in a major complication.

a. What is the structure shown?
b. What other structures can be damaged by ENT surgeons in the sinuses, leading to major complications?

43. This is the CT scan of a 23-year-old man who was punched in the right eye. Following the injury he complained of double vision.

a. What does the CT scan show and by what name is this particular injury usually known by?
b. What is the treatment for the man's double vision?

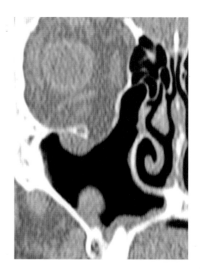

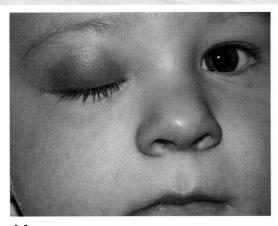

44. This is a 2-year-old child with a 3-day history of swelling around the right eye following an upper respiratory tract infection.

a. What is the diagnosis?
b. What is the cause of this condition?
c. What is the treatment, and what would the natural history of the condition be if untreated?

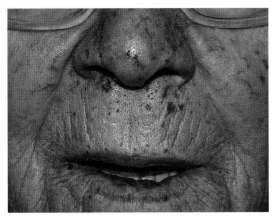

45. This is a photograph of an 80-year-old man suffering with recurrent epistaxis requiring repeated admission to hospital. His son, daughter and brother also have the condition.

a. What is the condition?
b. What is the mode of inheritance?
c. What is the treatment of the epistaxis associated with this condition?

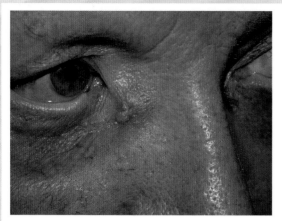

46. This 74-year-old woman has a discharging sinus close to her right eye. She also complains of a watery right eye.

a. What is the most likely diagnosis?
b. What is the appropriate treatment?

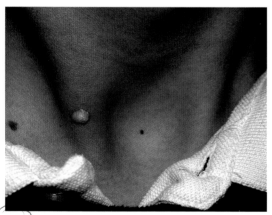

47. This 14-year-old boy presented with a lesion in his neck that had been discharging purulent material since early childhood.

a. What is the diagnosis?
b. What is the treatment?

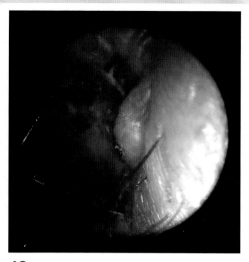

48. This is an endoscopic photograph showing a lesion in the nasal vestibule of a 24-year-old man. The man has similar lesions on his fingers.

a. What is the lesion?
b. What is the aetiological agent?
c. Is the lesion pre-malignant?
d. What is the treatment?

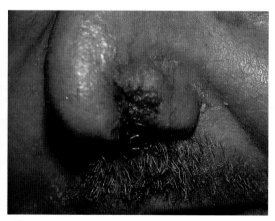

49. This is a photograph of a 70-year-old man with a lesion of the external nose.

a. What is the differential diagnosis?
b. What is the treatment?

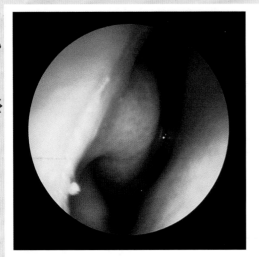

50. This is an endoscopic photograph of the nasal cavity of a 19-year-old man who suffers with nasal symptoms during the summer months in the UK.

a. What does the photograph show?
b. What is the likely diagnosis and what are the likely causative factors?
c. What is the treatment?

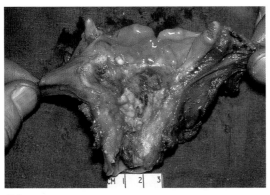

51. This photograph is of a surgical resection specimen.

a. What is the structure and disease demonstrated?
b. What is the aetiology of this disease?
c. How does it usually spread?
d. What treatment modalities are appropriate for it?

52. This is the ulcerated pinna of a 75-year-old man.

a. What is the likely pathological diagnosis?
b. Left untreated, how is the disease likely to progress?
c. What modes of treatment are appropriate?
d. What is the probable aetiology?

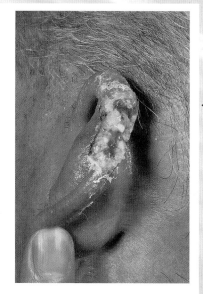

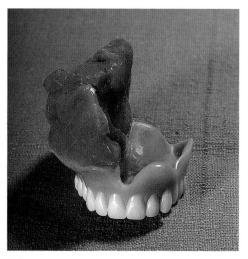

53. This prosthesis consists of a dental plate and obturator.

a. What procedure has the patient undergone?
b. What is epiphora?
c. Do such lesions usually present early or late?

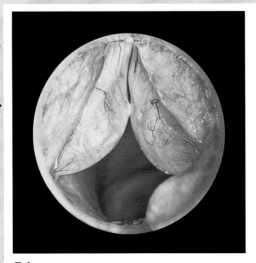

54. This is the endoscopic appearance of the larynx of a 44-year-old woman.

a. What is this a typical example of?
b. What are the possible aetiologies?
c. How would you treat the condition?

55. A 65-year-old pipe-smoker is worried about the appearance of his tongue.

a. What is the diagnosis and its cause?
b. Is the condition serious?
c. How is it treated?
d. How do tongue cancers usually present?

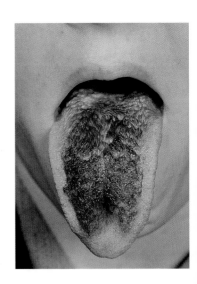

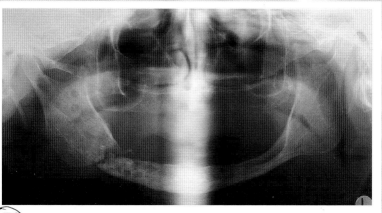

56. This is an X-ray of the mandible of a man who presents with an ulcer adjacent to the right lower alveolus.

a. What type of X-ray is this?
b. Why is it particularly useful?
c. What does it demonstrate in this instance?
d. If a biopsy demonstrates a malignancy would radiotherapy be an appropriate treatment?

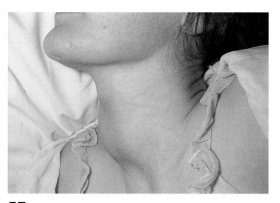

57. A 37-year-old lady presents with a year's history of a midline neck swelling.

a. What is the probable cause?
b. Is the underlying process likely to be benign or malignant?
c. How would you investigate the problem?
d. What particular symptoms would you ask about?

58. This patient has a vascular malformation of the skin of the right cheek.

a. What syndrome does this almost certainly form part of?
b. What are its other facets?
c. What are the resulting symptoms?

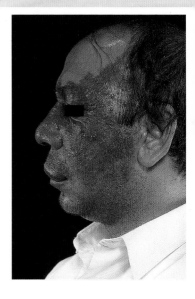

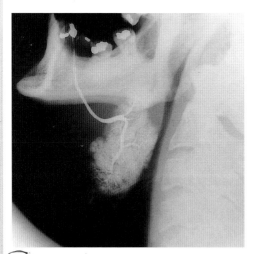

59. This is the X-ray of the oral cavity and upper neck of a 50-year-old man.

a. What investigation is being undertaken?
b. What are the likely symptoms necessitating it?
c. What specific abnormalities can the test demonstrate?
d. What nerves lie in close proximity to the structure?

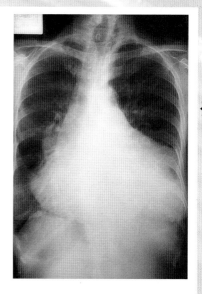

60. This is the chest X-ray of a 76-year-old man with a hoarse voice.

a. What is the disease process?
b. Why is he hoarse?
c. What other symptoms should be sought?
d. What is the treatment of these symptoms?

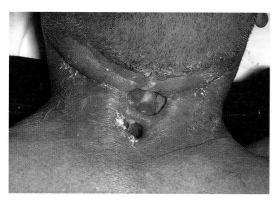

61. This man underwent a laryngectomy for advanced cancer three weeks prior to this photograph. There are two distinct 'holes' in the neck skin.

a. What is the lower one?
b. With what structure does the upper one probably communicate?
c. Which particular patients are at risk of such wound breakdown following major head and neck surgery?

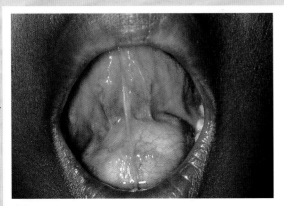

62. This lady has a swelling of the floor of her mouth.

a. Clinically how would you decide whether it was solid or cystic?
b. What investigation would be most helpful?
c. Are there any specific complications which can result from swellings at this site?

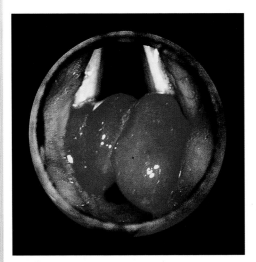

63. Prolonged endotracheal intubation can result in vocal cord damage with hoarseness and airway compromise following extubation.

a. What is the pathological process involved in this instance?
b. How can this situation be avoided?
c. How is it best treated?

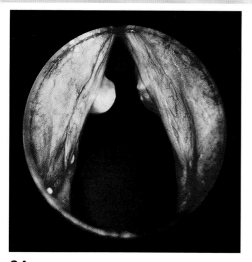

64. This is the larynx of a 45-year-old non-smoking schoolteacher.

a. What is the diagnosis?
b. How is it treated?
c. How can it be avoided?

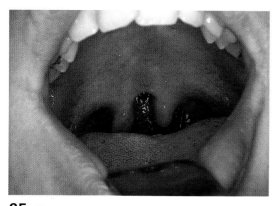

65. This is the appearance of the oropharynx of a boy with a history of nasal obstruction.

a. What does this slide demonstrate?
b. What could this be associated with?
c. Are there any surgical procedures that should be avoided?

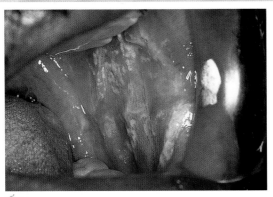

66. This is the appearance of the buccal mucosa of a 55-year-old female.

a. What is the clinical condition?
b. How would you confirm the diagnosis?
c. What is the treatment?

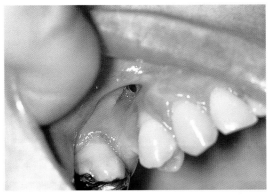

67. Following dental surgery this patient complains of foul-tasting debris intraorally along with right nasal symptoms.

a. What is the cause of the symptoms?
b. How would you investigate it further?
c. What is the treatment?

68. This is the cervical spine X-ray of a patient treated by radiotherapy for a laryngeal cancer.

a. What is the condition demonstrated?
b. What is the differential diagnosis?
c. How would you manage the patient?

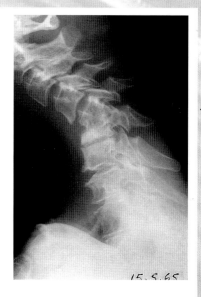

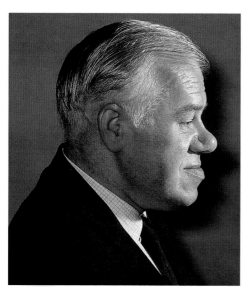

69. This man presents with hypertension and diabetes mellitus.

a. What is the clinical diagnosis?
b. How would you confirm this?
c. What treatment options are there?

70. This is the barium swallow X–ray of a patient with swallowing difficulties.

a. What is the descriptive term of the condition seen?
b. Will the patient find it easier to swallow fluids or solids?
c. In what other way might it present acutely?
d. What are the treatment options?

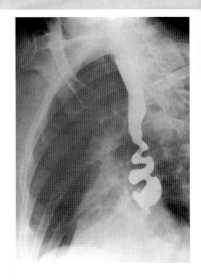

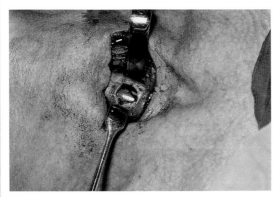

71. This surgical procedure is being undertaken for a patient with upper airways obstruction.

a. What surgical procedure does this demonstrate?
b. What are the indications for the operation?
c. Are there specific precautions that should be undertaken when undertaking the operation in young children?

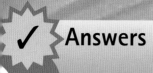

✓ Answers

1. *a.* The three holes in her lobule are man-made ear piercings.
   b. The anterior hole is a congenital pre-auricular sinus, which has become infected. Initially treatment should be with antibiotics. Sometimes abscesses can form, which may require drainage. In the long term surgical excision should be offered, although meticulous removal is required to prevent recurrence.

2. *a.* The use of a cotton-tipped applicator is not a good way to remove wax from the ear. The shape of the applicator makes it more likely to push wax and debris further down the external auditory canal, increasing a sensation of blockage.
   b. Wax (cerumen) does not have to be removed from the external auditory canal. The epithelium on the tympanic membrane and deep ear canal produces keratin debris, which is carried outwards by a natural active migratory process. Cerumen is produced by glandular secretion in the outer canal and is usually discharged naturally with the migrating keratin debris.
   c. Cotton-tipped applicators in the ear can cause a number of problems and should be strongly discouraged. They push the wax further down the ear canal, where it can become impacted on the tympanic membrane. They can damage the skin of the canal and cause otitis externa. If pushed too far down the canal they can rupture the tympanic membrane and in extreme cases cause injury to the ossicles and inner ear.

3. *a.* The lesion is a sebaceous cyst.
   b. Surgical excision would be most appropriate. This can usually be performed under local anaesthetic. Care has to be taken to remove all of the epithelial lining, otherwise the cyst can recur.

4. *a.* The photograph shows a 'cauliflower ear', caused by repeated injury to the pinna. A haematoma of the pinna strips the underlying cartilage of its blood supply, with ensuing cartilage necrosis and cosmetic deformity.
   b. The patient has had otitis externa with cellulitis spreading on to the face. A bacterial infection is most likely.
   c. The facial cellulitis should be treated with antibiotics, which may have to be given intravenously for severe infections. The underlying otitis externa should be treated with aural toilet and a local medication, usually an antibiotic/steroid combination.

5. *a.* The photograph shows congenital atresia of the external auditory canal.

b. When unilateral, usually no treatment is required for hearing as the opposite ear is often normal. Attempts to surgically re-establish the external auditory canal and middle ear in the past had very poor results and have been abandoned. In bilateral cases treatment is usually insertion of a titanium implant allowing attachment of a bone-anchored hearing aid (BAHA).

6.   a. The photograph shows stenosis of the deep part of the external auditory canal, occluding the tympanic membrane. The condition is sometimes called a 'false fundus' as the appearance can suggest that the tympanic membrane is more laterally placed than normal.

b. The condition arises from recurrent or chronic otitis externa. With persistent inflammation, the underlying skin becomes thickened, eventually resulting in a complete stenosis.

c. Treatment is very difficult once stenosis has occurred. Attempts can be made to reconstruct the auditory canal with skin grafts or to remove the stenosis with a laser. However, recurrence following surgery is common.

7.   a. The dressing is known as a Merocel™ Oto-Wick and is used in the treatment of otitis externa.

b. This material has the ability to expand when hydrated. On the left is the wick in its dry form, and on the right the hydrated version. This dressing is particularly useful in cases where swelling of the external auditory canal wall makes it difficult to use topical ear drops. After insertion of the Oto-Wick the drops can be put directly on to the wick, which will then expand and lessen the canal oedema.

8.   a. The photograph shows multiple exostoses of the external auditory canal. These can interfere with the natural skin migration within the canal, leading to accumulation of debris and otitis externa.

b. These lesions are sometimes known as 'swimmers exostoses'. They are thought to arise from repeated exposure of the auditory canals to cold water, and are hence often found in swimmers, surfers and scuba divers.

c. Individual episodes of otitis externa should be treated with aural toilet and topical antibiotic/steroid drops. For persistent cases with marked exostosis formation the hard areas of prominent bone can be drilled down and the canal widened.

9.   a. The correct method of examination is shown on the right. The external auditory canal is S-shaped and has to be straightened in order to obtain the best view of the tympanic membrane. This is achieved by gentle upward and outward traction on the pinna. In addition, in the picture on the left the otoscope is being held in an unwieldy manner in which it is more difficult to exhibit the fine control needed to avoid trauma to the external auditory canal.

10. *a.* The Rinne test.

   b. The Rinne test compares the responses to hearing by air and bone conduction. In a normal ear hearing by air conduction is more efficient than bone conduction and the tuning fork is heard better in air next to the ear (a positive Rinne test). In significant conductive deafness due to middle ear disease the tuning fork is heard better by bone conduction behind the ear (a negative Rinne test). In an ear with total sensorineural deafness bone conduction will be transmitted across the skull, giving a false-negative Rinne test.

   c. 512 Hz. Tuning forks below this frequency produce vibrotactile responses, while those above this frequency produce a sound that decays too quickly to produce a meaningful test.

11. *a.* The Weber test.

   b. In sensorineural deafness the tuning fork is heard predominantly in the better ear. In conductive deafness where the inner ear function is normal the tuning fork is heard predominantly in the worse ear. Using a combination of the Rinne and Weber tests the nature of deafness in a particular case can be diagnosed before confirmation by pure tone audiometry.

12. *a.* Testing for evoked otoacoustic emissions (OAE), sometimes known as 'cochlear echoes'.

   b. Otoacoustic emissions are sounds produced by the cochlea, which can be detected by sophisticated equipment placed in the external ear canal and linked to a computer. The presence of an evoked otoacoustic emission in response to a sound stimulus is a good indicator of normal cochlear function. Universal neonatal hearing screening is used to detect deafness at an early stage. The earlier significant deafness is detected the earlier appropriate rehabilitation can be given. In this way the chances of developing optimum speech and language development can be maximized.

13. *a.* The photograph shows an abutment for a bone-anchored hearing aid (BAHA). A screw fixture has been inserted into the skull behind the ear. The overlying skin and subcutaneous tissue has been removed and replaced with a non-hairy skin graft.

   b. BAHAs are used in people who cannot wear a conventional hearing aid in the external ear canal. This may be because of congenital atresia of the canals, recurrent discharge due to chronic otitis externa, or chronic otitis media. Sound impulses are conducted directly via the BAHA to the cochlea by bone conduction.

14. *a.* The principal risk is of noise-induced deafness with exposure over a prolonged period of time. The degree of deafness in an individual depends on the loudness of the noise, duration of exposure and individual susceptibility. Musicians are at risk when positioned close to loudspeakers.

b. The symptoms are insidious. At first there maybe deafness and tinnitus, which initially is reversible (temporary threshold shift). After repeated exposure permanent deafness and tinnitus may occur.

c. Once permanent deafness has occurred the hearing cannot be restored. In severe cases a hearing aid maybe useful. Minimization of future noise exposure is vital.

15. a. An Epley particle-repositioning manoeuvre, used in the treatment of benign paroxysmal positional vertigo (BPPV).

b. It is thought that BPPV is due to debris collecting in the vestibular labyrinth, usually the posterior semicircular canal, and stimulation of the canal ampulla. The aim of the Epley manoeuvre is to move the head in order to encourage the debris to flow away from the posterior canal into the vestibule of the inner ear, where it no longer causes a problem.

16. a. The function of the facial nerve.

b. The facial nerve travels from the brainstem through the temporal bone to branch in the parotid gland. The nerve is hence at risk during temporal bone skull base surgery, mastoidectomy and parotidectomy, and is monitored during these operations. The marginal mandibular branch of the facial nerve is also at risk during surgery of the submandibular salivary gland.

c. The facial nerve monitor detects electrical activity in the facial muscles in response to manipulation of the facial nerve. This activity is abolished by neuromuscular blocking agents used to produce paralysis during anaesthesia. These drugs must therefore be used with caution during facial nerve monitoring.

17. a. The clue is in the size of the external auditory canal, which is abnormally large. The patient has had an open cavity mastoidectomy performed which includes a meatoplasty to widen the ear canal. With a very wide ear canal obtaining the close fit required for a hearing aid to work may be a problem. In addition, some mastoidectomy cavities discharge, which would also hinder hearing aid use.

b. The patient is wearing a bone-anchored hearing aid (BAHA) attached to a titanium fixture inserted into the bone of the skull.

18. a. A serous effusion in the middle ear with a fluid level.

b. Nasopharyngeal carcinoma with secondary spread to the cervical lymph nodes. The middle ear effusion is caused by obstruction of the Eustachian tube.

c. Nasopharyngeal carcinoma is common in those of Chinese origin. Epstein–Barr virus has been implicated in the aetiology.

d. The middle ear effusion can be treated with ventilation tube insertion. A biopsy needs to be taken of the nasopharynx to confirm the diagnosis of carcinoma. Treatment is then usually a combination of radiotherapy and cytotoxic chemotherapy, with surgery for residual neck disease.

19. *a.* The photograph shows retraction of the tympanic membrane in the anterior part of the pars tensa and the superior attic regions. This type of retraction where the drum is very thin is often mistaken for a perforation. Careful inspection, however, usually reveals the thin membrane. In addition there is a possible effusion seen behind the drum anteriorly.

b. This appearance is the result of poor Eustachian tube function. In earlier childhood repeated insertions of ventilation tubes (grommets) may have been undertaken.

c. Current management depends on the symptoms. If the degree of deafness is mild and the opposite ear is normal no treatment is required. If deafness is a problem then a hearing aid could be contemplated. Some surgeons would advocate reconstructive surgery, arguing that the retraction of the drum can subsequently develop into cholesteatoma.

20. *a.* Insertion of a ventilation tube or grommet in the tympanic membrane.

b. Ventilation tubes are inserted for otitis media with effusion (OME/glue ear).

c. OME usually presents with conductive deafness. Children can have problems at school and poor speech development. One alternative to ventilation tubes is the use of hearing aids. Also, some advocate the use of an Otovent – this is basically a nasal balloon-blowing device aimed to improve Eustachian tube ventilation. In addition adenoidectomy performed at the same time as ventilation tube insertion can reduce the recurrence rate.

d. The child can swim. There is no need for earplugs with swimming pool water and sea water, as the surface tension effect prevents water from entering the middle ear. Soapy water lowers surface tension and is irritant. For this reason ENT surgeons usually recommend the use of cotton wool with petroleum jelly to plug the ears during shampooing and showering.

21. *a.* The photograph shows a ventilation tube (grommet) that has been naturally extruded from the tympanic membrane. There is a residual perforation in the anterior part of the drum, where the tube was originally positioned.

b. Following extrusion of ventilation tubes the residual perforation heals spontaneously in about 95% of cases. The extruding tube will be carried along the external auditory canal by the natural process of epithelial migration. Eventually the tube will become mixed with the wax in the outer part of the canal and usually fall out of the ear.

22. *a.* The photograph shows a granular area in the anterior part of the tympanic membrane – a condition known as 'granular myringitis'. The area represents localized infection, the onset and aetiology of which is often obscure.

b. The most common symptom is purulent discharge from the ear, which may be persistent or intermittent.

c. Many cases respond to local treatment with topical antibiotic/steroid drops or ointment. The use of local chemical cautery with silver nitrate can also be successful. Some cases are very resistant to treatment. In the most severe cases excision of the affected segment and grafting as in a myringoplasty operation may be required.

23. a. Traumatic perforation of the posterior part of the tympanic membrane. The symptoms depend on the degree of trauma. Most cases present with mild deafness, tinnitus and blood-stained discharge from the ear. If the ossicular chain is damaged the deafness will be more severe. In the most severe cases the inner ear can be traumatized, with leak of perilymph from the oval or round windows accompanied by sensorineural deafness and vertigo.

b. Most traumatic tympanic membrane perforations heal spontaneously within a few weeks. It is important to keep the ear dry. Antibiotic prophylaxis is not necessary. For the uncommon case in which healing does not occur, surgical repair with a myringoplasty operation may be required.

24. a. A discharging central perforation.

b. The most common infective agents are Gram-negative organisms such as *Pseudomonas* spp. and *Proteus* spp.

c. The most effective treatment is antibiotic/steroid ear drops. Most antibiotic ear-drop preparations contain aminoglycosides such as gentamicin and present a small risk of inner ear ototoxicity. This small risk, however, is outweighed by the risk to the inner ear of continued purulent infection. An alternative is to use drops containing quinolone preparations such as ofloxacin. Broad-spectrum oral antibiotics are usually ineffective. If the perforation persists, surgical closure with a myringoplasty operation may eventually be necessary.

25. a. A postauricular fistula between the mastoid air cells and the skin, with abscess formation.

b. Cholesteatoma. In developing countries where access to specialized ENT care is poor, chronic middle ear disease often presents at a late stage. Life-threatening intracranial complications of cholesteatoma are also more common.

26. a. The photograph shows a white structure in the posterior–superior part of the pars tensa of the tympanic membrane. Diagnostic possibilities characterized by their white appearance are cholesteatoma, tympanosclerosis and artificial replacement ossicles. In fact this particular white structure is a replacement ossicle made from synthetic hydroxyapatite.

b. The patient has hence undergone an ossiculoplasty operation. These operations are designed to restore the continuity of the middle ear ossicular chain and hence restore hearing. Ossicular discontinuity usually arises as a result of previous middle ear infection and is often associated with cholesteatoma. The commonest defect is loss of the long process of the incus, in which case a prosthesis can be inserted between the stapes head and drum or malleus. Loss of the stapes arch requires a prosthesis to be inserted between the stapes footplate and the drum, the results of which are often disappointing.

27. a. A dry central perforation of the tympanic membrane.
b. Conductive deafness.
c. (1) Size and position of the perforation. The larger the perforation the greater the deafness – posterior perforations are associated with greater deafness because they lie over the round and oval windows.
(2) Associated ossicular discontinuity – erosion of the incus long process or the stapes arch are associated with greater deafness.
(3) Active discharge – a wet ear is deafer than a dry ear.
(4) Tympanosclerosis can cause fixation of the ossicles and immobility of the tympanic membrane remnant.

28. a. Cholesteatoma in the pars flaccida or attic region of the tympanic membrane.
b. Cholesteatoma has the ability to erode bone. In the middle ear and mastoid this can result in facial nerve paralysis and erosion into the inner ear, causing suppurative labyrinthitis. Spread outside the temporal bone can cause intracranial complications such as meningitis, intracranial abscess and lateral sinus thrombosis.
c. A mastoidectomy operation. There are various techniques, which all aim to remove the cholesteatoma and restore a dry, safe ear.

29. a. The right ear is more prominent than the left. The appearance is otherwise normal.
b. The differential diagnosis includes a congenitally prominent ear, acute mastoiditis and acute otitis externa with postaural lymph nodes. In this particular case the diagnosis was acute otitis externa.
c. History and examination will usually reveal the diagnosis. In acute mastoiditis and otitis externa there will be earache with possibly discharge and deafness. In acute otitis externa traction on the pinna will be painful. In some cases where the diagnosis is difficult a CT scan of the temporal bone may be required, particularly where a cortical mastoidectomy may be required.

30. a. The photograph shows discharge in the deep ear canal. There is reddish granulation tissue at the junction of the ear canal and the tympanic membrane (tympanic annulus) in the posterior–superior part. The appearance is suggestive of underlying cholesteatoma in the posterior marginal region of the middle ear, with possible spread into the mastoid posteriorly.
b. It is likely that acute mastoiditis has arisen.

c. If a postauricular abscess is present surgical drainage is needed. Postaural cellulitis without abscess may respond to intravenous antibiotics. Underlying cholesteatoma will require mastoidectomy surgery.

31. a. A dry posterior perforation of the left tympanic membrane.
b. In the left of the picture the handle of the malleus can be seen. The perforation itself overlies the incudo–stapedial joint. The white structure passing horizontally across the perforation is the tendon of the stapedius muscle.

32. a. A nasal drop preparation containing a steroid, in this case betamethasone.
b. In order to reach the upper parts of the nasal cavity and ethmoidal regions.
c. Nasal polyposis.
d. The main danger is systemic absorption of steroid medication and adrenal suppression. This is a particular risk of intranasal betamethasone treatment, which as a result is limited to a maximum of 6 weeks at a time.

33. a. The photograph shows that the left eye is at a lower horizontal level than the right. The axis of vision for the left eye is abnormal, hence the diplopia.
b. The CT scan shows opacity of the ethmoid and frontal sinuses. In addition there is a cystic collection in the lateral part of the left frontal sinus, known as a mucocele, caused by obstruction to frontal sinus outflow. Although the mucocele is a benign condition, pressure erosion of adjacent bone can occur. In this case the bone forming the roof of the orbit has been eroded, with downward displacement of the globe, and resulting diplopia.

34. a. The symptoms of nasal stuffiness and purulent nasal discharge are suggestive of chronic sinus infection. Occasionally chronic infection of the frontal sinus can erode through the skin, resulting in a cutaneous fistula. Chronic sinus infections can also on rare occasions erode the bone protecting the anterior cranial fossa and present with intracranial complications such as meningitis and intracerebral abscess.
b. The nasal cavity should be examined to look for evidence of sinus infection. A CT scan should be obtained to define the extent of sinus disease and exclude intracranial complications. In this case surgery will probably be needed in order to re-establish sinus drainage, and also to remove the fistula.

35. a. Kaposi's sarcoma.
b. Most Kaposi's sarcoma lesions are asymptomatic and no treatment may be required. If cosmetically unsightly the lesions may be excised. Kaposi's sarcoma will also respond to radiotherapy or chemotherapy.

Treatment of the underlying HIV infection with anti-retroviral agents will also produce resolution of Kaposi's sarcoma.

36. *a.* Quadrilateral cartilage anteriorly, vomer bone posteriorly and the perpendicular plate of the ethmoid bone superiorly.

b. Olfactory filaments. The olfactory mucosa is specialized epithelium lying in the roof of the nasal cavity. The epithelium mediates the sense of smell. Odours passing into the nose stimulate receptors in the olfactory epithelium. Olfactory filaments then pass through small holes in the cribriform plate part of the ethmoid bone. These filaments then combine to form the olfactory nerves (the first cranial nerves), which run in the floor of the anterior cranial fossa into the olfactory cortex.

37. *a.* A malignant tumour of the nasopharynx. The two common tumours are squamous carcinoma and lymphoma. Nasopharyngeal carcinoma is particularly common in the Chinese community in south east Asia, where it is one of the most prevalent malignant diseases. It is thought to be related to Epstein–Barr virus infection.

b. The neck lump would be highly suspicious of a metastatic lymph node. Diagnosis could be confirmed by fine-needle aspiration for cytology. Blockage of the Eustachian tube by a nasopharyngeal malignancy causes deafness by production of a middle ear effusion.

38. *a.* The photograph shows a unilateral nasal polyp. The polyp has caused some expansion of the right nasal cavity. There is evidence of recent bleeding.

b. With unilateral nasal polyps neoplasia must be suspected. The commonest nasal neoplasm is the benign inverted papilloma. Malignant nasal neoplasms are rare but often have a poor prognosis. Examples are malignant salivary gland tumours, melanoma, squamous carcinoma and olfactory neuroblastoma. Sinonasal adenocarcinoma is more common in workers employed in the hardwood industry. In this particular case the other possibility is that the patient actually has bilateral simple polyps, with the right side being more severely affected.

c. Symptoms suggestive of malignancy include blood-stained nasal discharge, facial swelling, diplopia, loose teeth and deafness due to middle ear effusion.

39. *a.* The photograph shows a stream of mucus passing from the nasal cavity into the nasopharynx. The symptom of 'catarrh' is ill-defined – most people describe excess mucus in the nasopharynx. Catarrh is also known as postnasal discharge (PND). The nasal cavity normally produces a large quantity of mucus from glands and goblet cells within the nasal lining. This mucus is carried towards the nasopharynx by the action of cilia, and is normally clear fluid. When there is infection in the nose or sinuses the nasal secretions can become thick and purulent.

b. The normal clear nasal secretions are physiological and difficult to abolish. If there is purulent secretion rhinosinusitis would have to be suspected and treated depending on the history and endoscopic findings.

40. a. The photograph shows a deviation of the anterior part of the nasal septum, also known as the columella. This part of the septum is composed of cartilage. The deviation may have resulted from a previous nasal injury. In many cases deviation takes place over many years, starting in childhood and slowly increasing with facial growth.

b. If the nasal blockage is troublesome a corrective surgical procedure called a septoplasty could be performed. In this procedure the cartilage is mobilized from its bony attachments and repositioned. Because cartilage has a 'memory' these operations are sometimes unsuccessful as the repositioned cartilage adopts its former position. If anterior septal cartilage is removed cosmetic nasal deformity with nasal collapse may occur.

41. a. The photograph shows a diffusely swollen tongue that appears to be filling the oral cavity. The acute onset suggests either an acute allergic reaction or an episode of angio-oedema (a disorder of the complement system).

b. The immediate concern is to secure the airway. If the nasal cavity is patent a nasopharyngeal airway could be inserted. With life-threatening severe upper airway obstruction naso-tracheal intubation or emergency tracheostomy may be needed.

c. In the acute situation 1:1000 adrenaline (epinephrine) and a corticosteroid such as dexamethasone would be useful, given by intravenous or intramuscular injection. In addition an antihistamine preparation such as chlorphenamine (chlorpheniramine) could also be given.

42. a. The optic nerve running in the lateral part of the sphenoid sinus. Damage to the optic nerve can cause blindness.

b. The ethmoid sinuses are also close to the anterior skull base, which if damaged can result in a leak of cerebrospinal fluid. Severe bleeding can rarely occur as a result of damage to the interior carotid artery. These complications, while rare, are well recognized.

43. a. The CT scan shows a defect in the bone of the orbital floor with partial prolapse of the orbital contents into the maxillary antrum. This injury is known as a 'blowout' fracture of the orbit.

b. Double vision can occur with this injury for two reasons. First, the downward prolapse of the orbital contents may cause malalignment of the orbital axis, which could be corrected by prosthetic repair of the orbital floor. Second, some of the orbital muscles may have become entrapped, requiring direct repair via an orbital exploration.

44. *a.* Orbital cellulitis.

    b. Cellulitis of the periorbital and orbital tissues can either result from local orbital infection or spread from the neighbouring sinuses.

    c. Usually the condition responds to a short course of intravenous antibiotics. In severe cases a CT scan may reveal underlying sinusitis, which may have to be surgically drained. Left untreated, some cases may progress to orbital abscess formation, with a risk of permanent blindness.

45. *a.* Hereditary haemorrhagic telangiectasia (Osler–Weber–Rendu syndrome).

    b. Autosomal dominant.

    c. These patients can often suffer with severe epistaxis requiring repeated hospital admission. The usual measures of nasal cautery and packing are often not effective. Many alternative types of treatment such as laser therapy, skin grafting of the nasal septum and surgical closure of the nostrils (Young's procedure) have been performed, but with limited success.

46. *a.* Muco-pyocele of the lacrimal sac, which has discharged through the skin to form a sinus. The underlying cause is blockage of the distal nasolacrimal duct in the lateral wall of the nasal cavity. Tears are not able to flow normally through the lacrimal sac into the inferior meatus of the nasal cavity. Infection of the lacrimal sac then occurs, known as dacryocystitis.

    b. The treatment is to ensure drainage of the lacrimal system into the nasal cavity by an operation known as a dacryocystorhinostomy or DCR. The bone of the upper lateral nasal wall is removed, creating a large ostium from the lacrimal sac into the nasal cavity near the middle turbinate. This procedure can be performed through an external incision or endoscopically through the nose.

47. *a.* Congenital branchial fistula. These result from failure of complete development of the branchial arch and cleft system in utero. This system is responsible for the development of most of the structures of the head and neck.

    b. This particular patient opted to leave the lesion alone. The lesion can be excised, although the surgery is often difficult as the internal track of the fistula can pass deeply into the neck and classically has a communication with the pharynx near the palatine tonsil.

48. *a.* A nasal papilloma (wart).

    b. Human papilloma virus (HPV).

    c. No.

    d. Surgical excision, although these lesions have a tendency to recur.

49. *a.* The two main diagnostic possibilities are squamous and basal cell carcinoma. Basal cell carcinoma tends to be slower growing. Squamous cell carcinoma can spread to regional lymph nodes.

b. Surgery or radiotherapy. Surgical treatment will require skin flap or prosthetic repair of any resulting defect.

50. a. The inferior turbinate in the nasal cavity. The lining mucosa is swollen, with clear mucus present.
b. Allergy to pollen (grass or tree). Other possible allergens are house dust mite or animal fur, although these would tend to cause year-round (perennial) symptoms.
c. Medications used for pollen allergy include antihistamines, nasal steroid sprays and disodium chromoglycate spray (mast cell stabilizer).

51. a. A laryngectomy specimen that has been opened anteriorly. It demonstrates a large mucosal ulcer, which is a squamous cell carcinoma.
b. The vast majority of laryngeal cancers occur in patients who have a history of smoking, commonly associated with significant alcohol intake.
c. Early-stage disease usually remains confined to the larynx. More advanced tumours may metastasize to the ipsilateral anterior triangle jugular chain lymph nodes. Systemic metastases are rare unless the loco-regional disease is very advanced.
d. In general terms, early-stage disease is treated with radiotherapy while advanced disease is treated by surgery.

52. a. This is almost certainly a squamous cell carcinoma.
b. The lesion will enlarge and infiltrate the rest of the pinna and then the adjacent temporal bone. Metastasis to the parotid or mastoid lymph nodes may also occur.
c. Radiotherapy or surgery is the treatment of choice. Radiotherapy results in less cosmetic disfigurement but may result in a non-healing ulcer, particularly if the tumour has caused cartilage exposure.
d. Prolonged exposure to sunlight.

53. a. A radical maxillectomy.
b. This term describes excessive watering of the eye caused by obstruction of the naso-lacrimal duct.
c. Sinus carcinomas usually present late on with symptoms related to involvement of adjacent structures. With regard to maxillary sinus tumours presentation can take the form of ipsilateral glue ear, epistaxis or development of a loose tooth.

54. a. Reinke's oedema.
b. Hypothyroidism, smoking or voice abuse.
c. Hypothyroidism needs to be excluded. When the oedema is marked the excess mucosa should be trimmed from the vocal cords and the patient referred for speech therapy. Advice must be given regarding cessation of smoking.

55. *a.* Black hairy tongue is due to the colonization of the tongue mucosa by certain non-pathogenic bacteria.

b. No. Although it causes a great deal of patient concern it is not serious and does not lead on to any other problems.

c. The condition does not need to be treated but gentle brushing of the tongue, e.g. with a toothbrush, can help. Antibiotics are not indicated.

d. Tongue cancers usually present with a local ulcer, which may be sore or painful. In a minority cervical lymph node metastases may be the presenting symptom.

56. *a.* An orthopantomogram (OPG).

b. It demonstrates the whole mandible and lower jaw dentition and allows comparison of the two sides. It avoids the superimposing of one ramus over the other as can occur with lateral X-rays.

c. Erosion of the horizontal ramus on the right side. This is almost certainly malignant in origin, because of its irregular outline.

d. Radiotherapy would be inappropriate in such a situation as it would be very unlikely to eradicate disease infiltrating the bone.

57. *a.* This patient almost certainly has a goitre.

b. Given the generalized enlargement of the gland it is likely to be benign in origin.

c. Ultrasound scan of the thyroid and thyroid function tests.

d. Symptoms of hypo- or hyperthyroidism, hoarseness or dysphagia.

58. *a.* Sturge–Weber syndrome (encephalofacial angiomatosis).

b. As well as a capillary or cavernous haemangioma occupying the distribution of one of the branches of the trigeminal nerve, there is a leptomeningeal angioma intracranially.

c. Epilepsy is common. The majority of patients survive many years, though often with mental defects and/or a hemiparesis.

59. *a.* Submandibular gland sialogram.

b. Pain and/or swelling of the submandibular gland, often in association with eating or drinking.

c. Chronic obstruction of the main gland duct, which is usually due to a stenosis or a stone.

d. The marginal mandibular branch of the facial nerve, the lingual nerve and the hypoglossal nerve.

60. *a.* Congestive cardiac failure.

b. Such cardiomegaly can cause pressure damage to the left recurrent laryngeal nerve and therefore a vocal cord palsy.

c. More important than the hoarse voice is the risk of aspiration of food or saliva with consequent aspiration pneumonia. The patient should therefore be asked about problems relating to swallowing.

d. Along with the management of the heart failure, consideration should be given to improving laryngeal competence, e.g. by a thyroplasty or Teflon injection of the ipsilateral vocal cord.

61.
a. This is the tracheostome.
b. The upper skin defect almost certainly communicates with the pharynx, forming a pharyngocutaneous fistula.
c. Those with previous nutritional impairment and those who have previously undergone radiotherapy to the neck tissues.

62.
a. By manual palpation.
b. An MRI scan would delineate the mass and its relation to other soft tissue structures in the neck.
c. Any floor of mouth swelling that has the potential to increase in size is a threat to the airway as postero-superior displacement of the oropharynx can cause obstruction.

63.
a. This patient has typical vocal cord granulomas. These characteristically occur in the posterior part of the glottis and result from pressure necrosis of the mucosa overlying the arytenoid cartilages.
b. If a patient is likely to require intubation for longer than 48 h, consideration should be given to the creation of a formal or mini tracheostomy.
c. The granulomas can be dealt with by laser vaporization but recurrence can ensue.

64.
a. This is the characteristic appearance of singer's nodules.
b. Early nodules can be reversed by appropriate speech therapy. Nodules as large as those demonstrated are best removed by microlaryngoscopy.
c. Improved speech hygiene.

65.
a. A bifid uvula.
b. A submucosal cleft in the posterior portion of the bony hard palate with a mild palatal dysfunction.
c. Adenoidectomy in young children should be avoided in such instances.

66.
a. Clinically this is leukoplakia, which in itself is not a pathological diagnosis. It is important to distinguish mucosal abnormalities from oral candidiasis.
b. Having excluded candida (the plaques of which can be removed with a swab) the underlying pathology can only be ascertained by incisional biopsy.
c. Biopsy usually demonstrates a degree of dysplasia of the mucosa. This may not require active treatment but if it is very severe (e.g. carcinoma in situ) then stripping or laser excision of the involved mucosa is required.

67. *a.* An oro-antral fistula.

b. An OPG X-ray will not only demonstrate the status of the teeth but will also identify any associated infection in the maxillary antrum.

c. The fistula can usually be closed using a local mucosal rotation flap. However, if there is evidence of an associated sinus infection then this will also need to be treated for a successful result.

68. *a.* This patient has osteomyelitis of the cervical spine.

b. A crush fracture or tuberculosis are also possible causes.

c. The spine needs to be stabilized by appropriate bone grafting.

69. *a.* Acromegaly.

b. By a glucose tolerance test, and failure to suppress growth hormone to less than 2 mU/l. A pituitary MRI scan should also be performed, preferably with gadolinium contrast enhancement.

c. The treatment of choice is surgery. The gland can be approached trans-sphenoidally. If this is not appropriate then the choice is between treatment with a somatostatin analogue and/or radiotherapy.

70. *a.* Corkscrew or nutcracker oesophagus.

b. This is a disorder of neuromuscular control of the oesophagus and the patient will have more difficulty swallowing fluids than solids.

c. With angina-like chest pain.

d. It is important to reassure the patient regarding their cardiac status. A calcium entry blocker (e.g. nifedipine) is often helpful. In rare cases a lower oesophageal myotomy can be beneficial.

71. *a.* Tracheostomy.

b. Upper airways obstruction, protection of the airway for laryngeal incompetence, prolonged intubation.

c. In very young children the carotid artery can be mistaken for the trachea. Aspiration of the contents through a fine-bore needle is a wise precaution before creating a window in the trachea. In children the trachea is of small diameter and a vertical slit with stay sutures, rather than an excised window, should be created for the stoma.

Index

Page numbers in *italics* refer to answers